Translational Neuroscience

A Guide to a Successful Program

Translational Neuroscience

A Guide to a Successful Program

Edited by

Edgar Garcia-Rill, PhD

Director, Center for Translational Neuroscience
University of Arkansas for Medical Sciences
Little Rock, AR, USA

WILEY-BLACKWELL

A John Wiley & Sons, Ltd., Publication

Library of Congress Cataloging-in-Publication Data

Garcia-Rill, Edgar.
  Translational neuroscience : a guide to a successful program / Edgar Garcia-Rill.
      p. ; cm.
  Includes bibliographical references and index.
  ISBN 978-0-470-96071-4 (pbk. : alk. paper)
  I. Title.
  [DNLM: 1. Neurosciences–methods.   2. Translational Research–organization & administration.   WL 20]
  362.196′80072–dc23

                                                                          2011035229

A catalogue record for this book is available from the British Library.

Printed and bound in Singapore by Markono Print Media Pte Ltd
1   2012

Dedication

This book is dedicated to my wife, Catherine, my soul mate of many years, who makes my life complete.

Contents

Color plates appear between pages 96 and 97.

Contributors

Amy Ballard, MEd
Director of Clinical Research, Center for Translational Neuroscience

Veronica Bisagno, PhD
ININFA-CONICET, University of Buenos Aires, Buenos Aires, Argentina

Roger Buchanan, PhD
State University, Jefferson, AR, USA

William E. Fantegrossi, PhD
Department of Pharmacology and Toxicology, College of Medicine, University of Arkansas for Medical Sciences, Little Rock, AR, USA

Edgar Garcia-Rill, PhD
Director, Center for Translational Neuroscience, University of Arkansas for Medical Sciences, Little Rock, AR, USA

Kevin Garrison, PT, PhD
Center for Translational Neuroscience, University of Arkansas for Medical Sciences, Little Rock, AR, USA
and
Department of Physical Therapy, University of Central Arkansas, Conway, AR, USA

Abdallah Hayar, PhD
Center for Translational Neuroscience, University of Arkansas for Medical Sciences, Little Rock, AR, USA

Mark Mennemeier, PhD
Center for Translational Neuroscience, University of Arkansas for Medical Sciences, Little Rock, AR, USA

Christine Sheffer, PhD
Center for Translational Neuroscience, University of Arkansas for Medical Sciences, Little Rock, AR, USA
and
College of Public Health, University of Arkansas for Medical Sciences, Little Rock, AR, USA

Francisco J. Urbano, PhD
IFIBYNE-CONICET, University of Buenos Aires, Buenos Aires, Argentina
and
Fellow of the John Simon Guggenheim Memorial Foundation

Richard Whit Hall, MD
Center for Translational Neuroscience, and Department of Pediatrics,
University of Arkansas for Medical Sciences, Little Rock, AR, USA

Charlotte Yates, PT, PhD, PCS
Center for Translational Neuroscience, University of Arkansas for
Medical Sciences, Little Rock, AR, USA
and
Department of Physical Therapy, University of Central Arkansas,
Conway, AR, USA

Preface

This book is intended as a guide for basic scientists, clinician scientists, departmental chairs, deans, and presidents of academic health centers who are contemplating the development of a translational neuroscience program. While many of the studies, core facilities, and other programs are designed for translational neuroscience, all of these can be amended to apply to almost any research area. There is little doubt that future public and state support will be accompanied only by real advances in health-care outcomes and in almost any area of medicine. One answer to that demand is the development of translational research efforts. The topic of translational neuroscience is catchy but elusive. It is defined in many ways, and most scientists "think" that they know what it means. Most scientists have few ideas about how to go about performing it. We have received numerous invitations to speak in order to describe how we set up our center, how it is organized, how we developed our core facilities, and how we designed our career development program and mentoring activities. In addition, examples of successful translational neuroscience research are few and far between. There is a definite need and desire for such information, not only because of the direction research is taking but also because of the new requirements from funding agencies. This affects how research is designed, how faculty is recruited, and how students are attracted.

The early chapters of this book describe the process of how to organize a center for translational neuroscience, how to facilitate the mentoring of clinician scientists, how to develop a career development program, and how to design core facilities that can serve multiple kinds of translational research projects. Later chapters provide examples of the types of translational research efforts that can be undertaken using transcranial magnetic stimulation (TMS), designing studies on drug abuse and other conditions, using electrophysiology on adults and children, undertaking research on spinal cord injury, applications to the field of neonatology, and community-based research using telemedicine. The final chapter provides implications for the future and describes a novel role for basic science departments and how translational neuroscientists can be trained. Much of the information supplied here applies to all kinds of translational research, not just neuroscience research.

Hopefully, both administrators and researchers will appreciate the information provided, not only because they can develop translational research efforts, restructure both clinical and basic departments, but also because they can frame their recruitment and retention efforts. In addition, medical and graduate students will learn about the field and begin the search for training programs, advisors, and research topics that will provide translational research training appropriate for the coming years.

Acknowledgments

A large measure of the credit for the success of our center must go to our faculty, including our young recruits and established scientists, as well as our excellent staff and students. It is the energy and enthusiasm of the young that drives our indefatigable efforts. I am very grateful for the contributions to this book by some of those faculty members.

Without the support of the National Institutes of Health, in particular, the National Center for Research Resources, which has funded our Center (P20 RR20146), and the National Institute for Neurological Disease and Stroke, which has supported my lab for so many years (R01 NS20246), none of these advances would have been made. Institutional support is an absolute necessity for the development of infrastructure related to translational research, and we have been fortunate to have such an encouraging administration.

The suggestions and edits to versions of the book by Justin Jeffryes at John Wiley & Sons, Inc. are very much appreciated.

Personally, my research career is guided by two principles amply substantiated in (1) a lecture by WK Clifford of University College, London, in 1876, entitled, "The Ethics of Belief," in which he proposed, "it is wrong always, everywhere, and for anyone, to believe anything upon insufficient evidence," and (2) recently verbalized by Sam Harris in a 2010 book entitled, "The Moral Landscape," in which he proposes: "The more we understand ourselves at the level of the brain, the more we will see that there are right and wrong answers to questions of human values."

1 A Brief History of Translational Neuroscience

Edgar Garcia-Rill

SOME RECENT HISTORY

According to an Institute of Medicine (IoM) report released on July 17, 2003, translational research and interdisciplinary approaches to care must be more strongly supported by both academic health centers and federal funding agencies [1]. "Academic Health Centers: Leading Change in the 21st Century" strongly advocated increased attention to translational research. The report pointed out that, although "the various forms of research are interrelated, they are typically conducted by different scientists and funded separately." This approach will have to change, stated the IoM Committee on the Roles of Academic Health Centers in the twenty-first century. "Increased coordination and collaboration will be required to meet growing demands for rapid improvements in health care and for a greater focus on the types of research that answer questions about what does and does not work." Interestingly, the impression among congressional leaders has been that the justification for doubling the National Institutes of Health (NIH) budget was tied to increased support for translational and clinical research. Related to the need for translational research is a disturbing national trend showing that MDs holding R01 awards decreased from 20% in 1982 to only 4% in 2002. R01 awards are individual research grants to support a discrete projects and is the most common grant mechanism at the NIH. We researchers, both basic and clinical, stand to lose legislative and public support for research if the current trend continues.

Congressional leaders, policy-makers, and the public at large are increasingly concerned that the scientific discoveries of the past are failing to be translated into tangible benefits to public health. The response has been a series of initiatives making translational research a priority. However, two blocks to translational research have been identified, a lack of translation of basic science discoveries into clinical studies (T1) and

Translational Neuroscience: A Guide to a Successful Program, First Edition. Edited by Edgar Garcia-Rill.
© 2012 John Wiley & Sons, Inc. Published 2012 by John Wiley & Sons, Inc.

from clinical studies into medical practice (T2) [2,3]. The definitions of T1 and T2 research are actually that (a) T1 research addresses the translation of basic science breakthroughs into clinical trials, mainly on human subjects, while (b) T2 research attempts to implement those clinical trial findings into everyday clinical practice, thereby optimizing current treatments, for example, deciding between two equivalent therapies that may differ in cost-effectiveness, or developing novel therapies based on the results of well-drafted clinical trials. In fact, there has been a call to emphasize T1 and T2 research in proportion to its ability to improve health [4]. Additional blocks have been identified, blocks to T3 research foil attempts to move evidence-based guidelines into health practice, through delivery, dissemination, and diffusion of research, and blocks to T4 research impair the evaluation of the "real-world" health outcomes of a T1 application in practice. The latter require improved outreach programs, with considerable activity using telemedicine and other community-based research approaches.

Typical T1 blocks to translational research include lack of willing participants, regulatory burdens, fragmented infrastructure, incompatible databases, and lack of qualified investigators [3]. Among the T2 blocks to translational research are career disincentives, practice limitations, high research costs, and lack of funding [3]. These issues will be addressed throughout this book, but, before going further, a common misconception is that translational research must proceed on a linear basis. There is considerable precedent to suggest that the linear approach to translational research, that is, proceeding from basic research on animals to clinical studies on humans, followed by clinical trials, and then applied studies, is not necessarily optimal. The lack of translation from animal research to clinical trials, the so-called T1 obstacle, suggests that a bottleneck exists at the transition between the huge amount of knowledge from basic studies to the trickle of clinically oriented research at present. However, this linear concept has been questioned, and one of the leaders in suggesting that we should consider this process as cyclical is Bill Crowley at Massachusetts General Hospital in Boston, MA. He has developed convincing examples of bedside to bench research, in which it is the genetic testing of individuals with genetic disorders that can drive the design and development of animal models on which can be tested novel therapeutic avenues, which can then be carried back to the bedside [5]. A better model for the progression from basic to clinical research and back is thus a cyclical model in which research can begin at various points in the cycle (Figure 1.1). Given the fact that performing translational research is indeed open-ended, the NIH has been careful to leave definitions open to interpretation. This is a wise position, allowing the field to employ brainpower and imagination to forge the future of translational research. The lack of pigeon holing of the meaning of translational research should be viewed as an opportunity rather than a limitation.

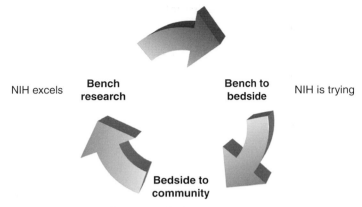

NIH excels   **Bench research**   **Bench to bedside**   NIH is trying

Bedside to community

Opportunity for improvement

Figure 1.1   Circular model of translational research. Research can begin at any point in the cycle and inform researchers about the needs of the preceding and subsequent processes. For example, an agent that derived from animal studies and was tested at the bedside may work well in a clinical trial, but bedside to community "real-world" applications may find it less effective. This would require amending the basic research and "recycling" in order to make a more efficient treatment.

In September of 2003, Elias A. Zerhouni, MD, the then new Director of NIH, presented his "roadmap" for medical research. "The purpose is to identify major opportunities and gaps in biomedical research that no single institute at NIH could tackle alone but that the agency as a whole must address to make the biggest impact on the progress of medical research." In reengineering the clinical research enterprise, "the exciting basic science discoveries currently being made demand that clinical research continue and even expand." "Translational research has proven to be a powerful process that primes the entire clinical research engine. Key to building a strong infrastructure will be to increase interactions between basic and clinical scientists, and ease the movement of powerful new tools from the laboratory into the clinic."

FUNDING TRANSLATIONAL RESEARCH

Academic health centers have been very good at making enormous strides in basic scientific research. In the coming years, this is likely to continue, but they will also need to begin refining the evidence base for health care. The general framework is that of discovery, which relies on basic research, followed by testing and application, which rely on clinical research, and then evaluation, which relies on applied research. Results from applied research are presumed to feed information to the formulation of further discovery. In reality, the process should begin at any point in the cycle.

Academic health centers will begin to explore this cyclic continuum, with those that redesign and plan properly being more successful at garnering NIH, and public, support. A number of obstacles exist to the transition toward this continuum of research activities. First, there is a low supply of clinical researchers; second, there is a lack of institutional organization to support translational research; and third, there are inadequate funding levels to support such research. The first obstacle will be addressed in the next chapter on mentoring of clinician scientists and how to set up a career development program. The second obstacle will be addressed in the last chapter on how academic health centers can reshape themselves to not only meet the challenges of translational research, but also take advantage of the wide-open field of possibilities available for performing translational research.

LACK OF FUNDING

The third obstacle is being met on one front with the development of the Clinical Translational Science Award (CTSA) program under the National Center for Research Resources (NCRR). Even before the General Clinical Research Center (GCRC) program at NCRR was revamped into the CTSA, NIH-wide initiatives were implemented. You may recall that the GCRC program was intended as an institutional facility for inpatient and outpatient research. That model was critically flawed in terms of being unable to facilitate research for young investigators and failed to provide sufficient training to increase the pipeline of clinical scientists. These deficiencies have been addressed in the design of the CTSA program. But, even before these changes, there were concerns about the low funding levels of clinically oriented research. For example, in the review of NIH applications, informal surveys at NIH determined that those applications that used animals tended to score on average 10 percentile points better than those that used humans. That is, simply the fact that the "human subject" instead of the "animal research" box on the face of the application was checked meant that, on average, these applications were scored at a lower level of enthusiasm. Of course, research on human subjects is in many ways more difficult to control, and more fraught with variability and technological difficulties, so that it is not hard to understand this attitude. In response, the review criteria of standard research grant applications were changed at all levels and institutes at NIH. The following are now typical review criteria, with the phrases in bold being the new ones added to accommodate the new emphasis on clinically oriented research. "*Significance*: Does this study address an important problem? If the aims of the application are achieved, how will scientific knowledge *or clinical practice* be advanced? What will be the effect of these studies on the concepts, methods, technologies, *treatments, services, or preventative interventions* that drive this field? *Approach*: Are the conceptual *or clinical framework*, design, methods, and analyses adequately developed, well integrated, well reasoned, and appropriate to the aims of the project? Does the applicant acknowledge potential problem areas and consider alternative tactics? *Innovation*: Is the project original and innovative? *For example*: Does the project challenge existing paradigms *or clinical practice*; address an innovative hypothesis or critical barrier to progress in the field? Does the project develop or employ novel concepts, approaches, methodologies, tools, or technologies for this area? *Investigators*: Are the investigators appropriately trained and well suited to carry out this work? Is the work proposed appropriate to the experience level of the principal investigator and other researchers? Does the investigative team bring complementary and integrated expertise to the project (if applicable)? *Environment*: Does the scientific environment in which the work will be done contribute to the probability of success? Do the proposed studies benefit from unique features of the scientific environment, *or subject populations*, or employ useful collaborative arrangements? Is there evidence of institutional support?"

Launched in 2006 and led by the NCRR, the CTSA program is working at institutional, regional, and national levels to create a discipline of clinical and translational science. Its primary mission is to more efficiently translate the rapidly evolving knowledge developed in basic biomedical research into treatments to improve human health. From 2006 to 2008, 38 academic health centers and research institutions in 23 states became part of the consortium. In 2010, the consortium consisted of 55 member institutions. When fully implemented, approximately 60 institutions will be linked in a way that is intended to energize the discipline of clinical and translational science with >$500 million per year of NIH funding. Diversity in the size, scope, and geographic location of participating institutions has been mandated because such diversity is thought to strengthen the CTSA consortium and enhance its impact.

More recently, the NIH Scientific Management Review Board voted on December 7, 2010, to approve a recommendation to newly appointed NIH Director Francis Collins to create a new NIH center focused on translational medicine and therapeutics called the National Center for Advancing Translational Science (NCATS). The proposed center would house the currently NCRR-administered CTSA program along with the Cures Acceleration Network, Molecular Libraries Program, Therapeutics for Rare and Neglected Diseases, and Rapid Access to Interventional Development, as well as new NIH-FDA partnership activities.

These changes have generated considerable concern in the research community, and it is not yet clear whether congressional support will follow. For example, one of the mandates of NCATS will be the development of new drugs for therapeutic use. This is a response to the disturbing reduction in the pharmaceutical industry of spending on research and development, all in the face of a decline in the output of new drugs approved by the Food and Drug Administration (FDA). While Dr. Collins has been predicting that gene sequencing will lead to a host of new treatments, investments in the billions of dollars by the drug industry have failed to yield new gene-related therapies. While the NIH has historically been very good at supporting basic research, many wonder how good it will be at drug development, which requires a different set of skills. On the plus side, it may turn out that such an effort may generate a new type of researcher who can perform in both academic and drug company settings. On the minus side, this is the first time in the 80-year history of the NIH that an institute will be dismantled and the parts scattered across the rest of NIH. Historically, orphan programs tend to be phased out of existence by the "host" institute. These concerns are likely to persist for years, but it is hoped that unbiased and independent assessment of the success of the NCATS will tell us if the investment is worthwhile.

There are additional concerns. For example, the creation of the several components of the NCATS will require most, if not all, of the funding accorded the NCRR in order to support these new directions. This means that cuts to other programs could ensue. Among the most controversial consequences of eliminating the NCRR is the future of such programs in the NCRR portfolio as the Research Centers for Minority Institutions that supports centers as the name implies, and the Institutional Development Award (IDeA) program that supports such statewide infrastructure development incentives as the IDeA Networks of Biomedical Research Excellence (INBRE) program, and the Centers of Biomedical Research Excellence (COBRE) program that underwrite the creation of thematic, multidisciplinary centers, all in states with historically low levels of Federal funding. These programs are intended to provide diversity and correct the geographical inequalities in research support. These fairly small programs produce a huge return on investment, and add to the economic impact of academic health centers in small and medium-sized communities, which is in the order of >$3 billion for an average medical school [1]. The ramifications of this reorganization are likely to have considerable and lasting impact.

MAKING NIH FUNDING MORE EQUITABLE AND EFFICIENT

Most of the research in academic health centers in the United States is done under the auspices of the NIH. The NIH budget is currently around $31 billion, which is about 0.27% of the Gross Domestic Product (GDP), and about one half of what most developed countries spend on research. It can be argued that we do not spend enough on research. On the other hand, the United States spends twice as much for health care per capita as other developed countries, yet lags behind other wealthy nations in such measures as infant mortality and life expectancy. This can be interpreted to mean that the way we distribute our research dollar does not have sufficient impact on health care. Moreover, as mentioned in the preceding text, there is a regional inequality in the funding of biomedical research, being concentrated on the two coasts. The top 10 institutions are awarded about a third of all NIH extramural funding, while the next 40 institutions receive over one half of all the grant money. Institutions in states that account for over 20% of the population receive less than 10% of all awards. The NIH has instituted a number of measures to improve medical research. For example, during the Clinton administration, the NIH budget was doubled over a 10-year period. This had the effect of funding much new research and attracting three times the number of scientists into research, but it also made grants not twice, but three times more competitive. In the meantime, the disparity between the "haves" and the "have-nots" grew more severe. Such programs as INBRE and COBRE are essential to developing diversity in facilities throughout the country, increasing areas of research excellence, and serving the needs of all taxpayers. This is especially true when the issue is one of improving health for the public at large.

One massive cost that has not been addressed but could save millions of dollars is the establishment of a national indirect cost rate. Indirect costs are subsidies to the institution holding an NIH award for expenses incurred by the facilities related to the performance of the award such as heat and air, cleaning, purchasing, human resources, accounting, regulatory oversight, and so on. That is, an institution with a 50% indirect cost rate that is granted a $1 million award will actually receive $1.5 million, $1 million in direct costs and $0.5 million in indirect costs. Unfortunately, many institutions have negotiated rates as high as 100% or more. The same $1 million award at one of those institutions would cost NIH $2 million or more for performing the same research project. A national indirect cost rate of, say, 40% would be a good starting point toward saving millions of dollars that could be used to implement more fundable research grant applications.

HOW MUCH FUNDING IS NEEDED?

While the current level of funding at $31 billion would seem impressive, lack of investment in research is much more expensive. The current NIH budget is divided into support for research grants (~85%) that includes backing for 50,000 awards and 325,000 scientists, support for the NIH intramural program (~10%), and pretty reasonable costs for administration (~5%). It is estimated that, for every dollar spent on research, it generates $2.1 dollars to the local economy in terms of creation of jobs for highly skilled workers, faculty salaries, and so on [1]. A report by the Joint Economic Committee of the United States Senate in 2000, entitled "The Benefits of Medical Research and the Role of NIH," estimated that publicly funded research in general generates high rates of return to the economy, averaging 25–40% per year [6]. Compare this rate of return to the corporate model, where corporations often use an expected rate of return of 15% as the minimum for considering investments. "Despite the great success of medical advances in reducing health care costs for many diseases, there is concern that new medical technologies continue to drive health care spending upward. Certainly, NIH funding has created an increased *supply* of new technologies for diagnosis and treatment. However, the main reason that health care costs have risen quickly is the prevalence of third-party payers in the US health care system. Third-party payment in its current form artificially increases *demand* for health care by reducing incentives to use cost-saving technology" [6]. A more recent Wellcome Trust report from 2008 studied the economic benefits of the United Kingdom's public and charitable investment in medical research [7]. The report concluded that the health and economic gains were equivalent to a 37% annual rate of return for mental health research *in perpetuity*. This analysis also found that the delay between research expenditures and health benefits was 17 years on average. They emphasized that shortening this time lag would improve the rate of return. Translational research is designed to accomplish just that. In the last chapter, we will discuss the benefits of translational research, and how academic health centers can reinvent themselves to regain the steadfast support of the public at large so necessary to the continued success of medical research.

There is also the danger of losing our leadership in biotechnology and medical research to countries that spend more of their GDP on biomedical research. This means that we need to fund research to the highest levels possible. What levels? When President Obama instituted the American Recovery and Reinvestment Act, an additional $10 billion dollars was thrown into the health care research pot. NIH and other agencies responded quickly to issue imaginative and purposeful requests for applications (RFAs). Some programs with 30 or so awards to make expected to receive a few hundred applications. They received thousands. In one case, a program that was to fund 300–400 grants received over 23,000 applications. These data suggest that there are currently enough meritorious applications to accommodate a $10 billion increase in the NIH budget. However, given the history of the doubling of the NIH budget in the 1990s, such increases should be implemented more gradually in order to account for the increased number of scientists and applicants. Unfortunately, only cuts to this budget are being contemplated, mortgaging our future further.

How does an agency review 23,000 applications instead of a few hundred? Usually, a review committee for individual investigator applications will convene 15–20 experts in the field, with each reviewing 5–6 applications, and most applications requiring three reviewers. Of the 60 or so applications considered by a committee, only a few will earn a fundable score. The review of thousands of applications would require thousands of reviewers. While many scientists consider performing NIH reviews to be a duty as a researcher and faculty member, an equal number avoid the work-load these reviews entail. Grant reviews are time consuming and difficult, requiring hours of reading per application on the part of the reviewer. The response of NIH to this complaint has been to reduce the length of the applications. Applications had a 25-page limit for many years, with about one half of the material representing experimental design and methods. Applications are now half that length. While this requires better writing on the part of the applicant, the brevity of the application places the applicant at a disadvantage since a reviewer can easily dismiss an application because it does not have enough "detail," especially in the methods. This is used by some reviewers, whether justified or not, to triage applications, with little chance of appeal or recourse, generating uncertainty about the review process.

The NIH has also reduced the review committee meetings from 2 days to 1 day. This decreases the amount of time each application is discussed. During the review, applications that used to be discussed at length are now discussed for 15–20 minutes, depending on the degree of differing opinions by reviewers. In 90% of cases, all three reviewers are pretty much on the same page, and their scores reflect the consensus. The shortness of the review, however, makes it more difficult to determine if a reviewer is actually correct in the assessment, and there is little time for insisting that reviewers justify their opinions. This introduces additional uncertainty about the review process.

For years, the NIH review committees functioned under a scoring system that allowed reviewers to assign scores from 1.0 (best) to 5.0 (worst) with decimal places, that is, 1.1, 1.2, and so on. Most reviewers tended to use only one half of the range and score most grants between 1.0 and 2.5, that is, they had a range of 25 possible scores. Because of the number of highly meritorious grant applications, fundable scores tended to cluster between 1.0 and 1.6, or even lower. Awards were made using a percentile calculation across multiple review committees, and funding percentiles were at about 20 or less. As funding became more difficult due to flat budgets, especially during the GW Bush administration, purchasing power decreased due to inflation, and competition increased. Scores became even more compressed, between 1.1 and 1.3 or less, while funding levels decreased to 10 or even lower percentiles. NIH then decided to change the scoring method, introducing a 1–9 scoring range using only whole numbers. As expected, most reviewers use only one half of the range, that is, 1–5, so that now there is a range of five possible scores. Therefore, the discrimination between grant applications has decreased by 80%, adding further uncertainty to the review process. While NIH administrators may believe that reviewers will ultimately find a happy medium and use the whole 1–9 range, the fact is that this did not happen for years using the 1.0–5.0 range of scores. The current scoring system simply may not be discriminating between the best and the best of the best.

However, it should be noted that the peer review process at NIH has worked well for many years, excellent science is still supported, and most scientists do trust the system. The problems cited represent issues that undermine trust and do need remediation, but the process in general does work and it works well. How do you fix these (given the larger picture, minor) problems? First, reviewers need to justify their opinions better, making it imperative that the chair and other members of the committee question apparently unsubstantiated opinions. Second, the issue of lack of detail in methodology should be granted only partial weight, especially if the applicant has published previously using the methodology. Third, a wider range of scoring should be used, the current system will only lead to frustration and undermine the credibility of the review process. The key is to create confidence that the review process is fair, which it is in the vast majority of cases. It is the overcritical nature of many reviewers that undermines the process, with less thought given to the implications and potential benefits of the research. Any application can be nit-picked to death, so that it is incumbent on administrators, chairs, and members of review panels to determine when this is happening and put a stop to it.

Funding for translational research needs to be unbiased and sufficiently critical to ensure its validity, but without retreating into the overused excuse that experiments on humans cannot be as well controlled as those on animals. The experience of the reviewers in this field will be critical in ensuring accurate reviews. In addition, RFAs and program announcements for funding should be less restrictive, allowing for circular models of translational research to be applied. Reviewers with "big picture," rather than "nit-picking," attitudes will be sorely needed. Knowledge of the great number of options available for performing translational research, some of which will be discussed in the following chapters, will be essential in determining which science should be funded.

MEDICAL RESEARCH FUNDING IN EUROPE

The level of Federal funding in Europe is <15% than that of the United States, although there are almost as many scientists [8]. While the NIH budget was being doubled, increases in Europe amounted to <25%. Much of the funding in Europe is dedicated to applied research, while most of the funding in the United States is dedicated to basic research. European research and development accounts for ~1.9% of the GDP in the larger countries, and much less in smaller, newer members of the European Union (EU) [8]. Most research in Europe is carried out in state universities, which are mainly supported by national and local governments. However, new initiatives are driving research in new directions. More attention is being paid to research by such entities as the Wellcome Trust Foundation in the United Kingdom, and declarations proposing an increase in the national investment for research to approach 3% of the GDP have been issued. In addition, the formation of a European Research Council (ERC) has been proposed, but current economic forces make it unlikely at this time.

Only ~€5 billion of the ~€50 billion research and development budget of the EU is dedicated to basic research [6]. Initiatives for translational research have yet to be implemented and funding allocated for such avenues. Funding from the EU as well as member nations need to be committed to an entity such as the ERC. Hopefully, the ERC can avoid some of the problems in the US funding mechanisms, keeping in mind that, despite the criticisms leveled at some of the mechanics, the fact is that the peer review system at NIH is an excellent example of fair and equitable scientific peer review. As in the United States, Europe faces an aging population, increasing rates of obesity, diabetes, mental health disorders and neurodegenerative diseases, rising allergic disease rates, and the daunting tasks of addressing cancer and cardiac disease. There is little doubt that scientific excellence and creativity are alive and well in Europe, witness the growing number of Lasker Award and Nobel Prize winners from the EU.

Initiatives for translational research in Europe lag behind those being implemented in the United States, mainly because of the lower level of support for basic research. However, Europe has a considerable base of clinical trials (mostly initiated from the United States), with a clinical trials network, the European Clinical Trials Network, and a new oversight agency similar to the FDA named the European Medicine Agency. Therefore, the transition to translational research should not be too difficult, given appropriate increases in support for medical research.

Specifically in the United Kingdom, the scientific research that is funded by the government is regulated by the Research Councils. Two research councils fund neuroscience research: the Medical Research Council (MRC) and the Biotechnology and Biological Sciences Research Council (BBSRC). Recent important changes in the grants schemes offered by the Wellcome Trust, one of the major funding sources for biomedical research in the United Kingdom, have produced an overload of applications to the MRC (and possibly the BBSRC). This has decreased the funding levels in the MRC to one of the lowest levels in recent times. This situation has been aggravated by recent funding cuts. In this scenario, one of the predictions is that attention will now shift to the funding opportunities from charities supporting research oriented to cure or advance the knowledge of specific neurological diseases. This may increase the awareness in the basic science community to produce research with more translational possibilities.

However, it is clear that there is insufficient pressure from the MRC to fund translational neuroscience, even though the MRC is committed to fund research with potential clinical applications. As with NIH, all grant proposals submitted to the MRC are required to identify the public and economic benefits as well as the specific potential for any given proposal to advance the medical knowledge and to provide therapeutic possibilities.

Although this has become mandatory in every application, many of these are without a clear strategic plan of how could this be achieved.

On the other hand, in the United Kingdom (as in the United States), some basic scientists consider that the funding opportunities for pure basic research are increasingly more restricted. Most of the funding needs to be justified in terms of immediate or medium-term benefits for the society. Thus, the lack of clear funding channels for distinct research purposes produces ambiguity in the scientific community with regard to the most appropriate sources of funding for distinct research programs. Separate funding channels for distinct types of research, from basic to translational to implementation in the community, may help to shape the priorities for each funding body and unclog those opportunities where translational neuroscience could most benefit.

Other efforts have been initiated during the education and training of new generations of medical doctors. Some UK universities encourage medical trainees to enroll in a laboratory and carry out a project for a variable period of time, usually no less than 3 months. This allows future generations to obtain first-hand experience at the bench and appreciate how basic science is carried out, closing the gap between basic science and clinical professionals.

In conclusion, there is room for improvement in the support of translational research in Europe. There is no systematic endeavor to bring together basic and clinical scientists, and this ends up being a matter of personal choice for each scientist rather than a program strategy. More efforts are needed to support that part of the scientific community that is able to translate basic research findings into therapeutic benefits, as is encouraged by privately funded organizations and universities across Europe.

It should be noted that Asian countries are investing in research and development at higher levels. While the GDP in China has doubled in the last 10 years, its investment in research is increasing dramatically to about one-third of the levels in the United States. As their GDP grows, so should their investment in research and development. However, it is unclear how much is devoted to basic research, since target areas, like stem cell research, are being funded disproportionately, and most funding is still for applied programs.

Despite the mostly negative news on the research enterprise, we know that the current downturn is tied to the economy worldwide. This downturn will doubtless be followed by an upturn, with a reestablishment of effective funding levels. The scientific community can hasten the return of solid support from funding agencies and governments at large if they help justify their efforts, and if they draft research that addresses the needs of the public health. A simple way to accomplish that is to place a premium on translational research. The perception is that for too long funding has been directed at curiosity-driven research, with less attention paid to the pipeline of new treatments and cures. We know that basic scientific research, especially brain research, is absolutely essential to the understanding of brain processes, and, therefore, necessary for the development of those cures. However, there is plenty of room for translational research that addresses immediate health care concerns. The more the funding agencies, governments, and the public at large are informed about these efforts, the faster proper support for all research efforts will return.

The next chapter will discuss T1 and T2 blocks to translational research and how these can be overcome through a mentoring and career development program, while the following chapter will describe how infrastructure, in the form of core facilities that meet translational research goals, can be developed. Following several chapters describing examples of translational research, the final chapter will discuss how basic science and clinical departments can develop novel interactions to optimize translational research. Such reorganization could take advantage of the new funding avenues available, all in order to help improve the health of the public, while maintaining preeminence in biomedical research in both the United States and Europe.

REFERENCES

1. Committee on the Role of Academic Health Centers in the 21st Century; Kohn LT, ed.; Academic Health Centers. (2004) Leading Change in the 21st Century. Institute of Medicine, National Academies Press, Washington, DC.
2. Crowley WF. (2003) Translation of basic research into useful treatments: how often does it occur? Am J Med 114, 503–505.
3. Sung NS, Crowley WF, Jr., Genel M, Salber P, Sandy L, Sherwood LM, Johnson SB, Catanese V, Tilson H, Getz K, Larson EL, Scheinberg D, Reece EA, Slavkin H, Dobs A, Grebb J, Martinez RA, Korn A, Rimoin D. (2003) Central challenges facing the national clinical research enterprise. JAMA 289, 1278–1287.
4. Woolf SH. (2008) The meaning of translational research and why it matters. JAMA 299, 211–213.
5. Seminara SB, Crowley FC. (2002) Genetic approaches to unraveling reproductive disorders: examples of bedside to bench research in the genomic era. Endocr Rev 23, 382–392.
6. Mack C. (Chairman of Joint Economic Committee of the United States Senate). (2000) The Benefits of Medical Research and the Role of NIH. http://www.faseb.org/portals/0/pdfs/opa/2008/nih_research_benefits.pdf.
7. Health Economics Research Group, Office of Health Economics, and Rand Europe. (2008) Medical Research: What's it worth? Wellcome Trust. http://www.wellcome.ac.uk/stellent/groups/corporatesite/@sitestudioobjects/documents/web_document/wtx052110.pdf.
8. Philipson L. (2005) Medical research activities, funding, and creativity in Europe. Comparison with research in the United States. JAMA 294, 1394–1398.

2 Mentoring in Translational Neuroscience

Edgar Garcia-Rill

This chapter includes a discussion of the process of carrying out human subject research, the bedrock of translational research, which is necessary for understanding how mentoring for translational neuroscience can be undertaken. It is first essential to consider the reasons behind T1 and T2 blocks to translational research so that we can design a system for overcoming those blocks. The definitions of T1 and T2 research were covered in the previous chapter but are worth reiterating. T1 research addresses the translation from basic science breakthroughs into clinical trials, mainly on human subjects, while T2 research attempts to implement those clinical trial findings into everyday clinical practice, thereby optimizing current treatments or developing novel therapies based on the results of well-drafted clinical trials. The typical T1 blocks to translational research include (a) lack of willing participants, (b) regulatory burdens, (c) fragmented infrastructure, (d) incompatible databases, and (e) lack of qualified investigators. Among the most common T2 blocks to translational research are (a) career disincentives, (b) practice limitations, (c) high research costs, and (d) lack of funding. We will first discuss each of these blocks and suggest potential solutions before delving more deeply into perhaps the most important solution to these blocks, the mentoring of more clinician scientists to facilitate their careers as independent investigators.

T1 BLOCKS

Lack of willing participants

This is a particularly difficult block to overcome. Access to human subjects with specific disorders would seem manageable; after all, participating in research that could help their condition would seem an advantage. Usually, subjects are recruited using flyers and ads strategically placed in areas

Translational Neuroscience: A Guide to a Successful Program, First Edition. Edited by Edgar Garcia-Rill.
© 2012 John Wiley & Sons, Inc. Published 2012 by John Wiley & Sons, Inc.

thought to be frequented by such potential subjects. The goal of recruitment efforts is to obtain access to a sufficient number of people since only a small portion of the group that is actually targeted will become an enrolled participant in a clinical project or trial. Greater numbers increase the likelihood of obtaining a large enough sample of people that will actually match a very specific set of inclusion and exclusion criteria that are usually required for participating. For example, having suffered a stroke may be a necessary qualification to be included in a trial, but the presence of seizures, or taking drugs that control seizures, may exclude one from the study. Abiding by a certain set of criteria is essential to extracting reproducible and meaningful data from a study; therefore, there is danger in loosening these restrictions. Since access to sufficient numbers is key, some studies on rare disorders may be doable only in large communities. On the other hand, smaller communities have a more positive attitude toward their medical centers, making them more likely to attract research subjects.

In order to support human research across a number of disorders, it will be essential to develop facilities focused on recruitment called Recruiting Core Facilities, with dedicated project managers who are familiar with local and regional medical populations. Such a facility will need to develop Web sites and telephone call-in centers to help recruit subjects. The use of databases of ongoing and past studies will be critical to accessing subjects for follow-up studies, for example, in tracking the long-term effects of low birth weight in teenagers and adults that were born premature 10 and 20 years before. Such studies could ask the question, how can we improve delivery and postnatal treatment to prevent long-term deficits in some of these patients? The implementation of such a Core Facility requires investment on the part of the Clinical Translational Science Award (CTSA) and/or academic health center because this type of asset will be essential to building the number and quality of human research programs at these institutions. Investigators will need to work with this centralized facility, in addition to implementing the usual recruitment tools, in order to optimize subject recruitment and speeding their research project.

Regulatory burdens

Perhaps the most daunting prospect for a new investigator is applying for approval of their human research project from the Institutional Review Board (IRB). The IRB, whose mandate is to protect the rights and safeguard the welfare of research subjects, is constituted by the institution or academic health center to review human research protocols, and its members include faculty from various colleges as well as lay members from the community. The details of this process are available at the National Institutes of Health (NIH) Web site for the Office of Human Subjects Research. Briefly, Federal law requires the Department of Health and Human

Services (DHHS) to issue regulations for the protection of human subjects of research and to implement a program of instruction and guidance in ethical issues associated with such research. These regulations are codified at Title 45, Part 46 of the Code of Federal Regulations, Protection of Human Subjects (45 CFR 46). They provide for the prospective review and approval of human subject research activities by an IRB, a committee whose primary mandate is to protect the rights and welfare of humans who are the subjects of research. The regulations also incorporate a number of ethical principles regarding all research involving human subjects as expressed in the report of the National Commission for the Protection of Human Subjects of Biomedical and Behavioral Research entitled The Belmont Report [1]. All institutions, including the NIH, which receive funds from the DHHS to conduct or support research with human subjects are subject to these regulatory requirements and are to be guided by the ethical principles of The Belmont Report. This report first addresses the differences between what constitutes research compared to research, then goes on to describe a series of ethical principles, namely, respect for persons, beneficence (basically doing no harm and maximizing possible benefits while minimizing possible harms), and justice (equally distributing benefits). The report spells out general principles to the conduct of research that involves the following requirements: informed consent, risk and benefit assessment, and the selection of subjects of research. These principles and requirements, which have grown in number and complexity since the report was developed, now guide the deliberations of IRBs throughout the country.

A medium-sized institution may need as many as three committees, each with 8–10 members meeting 2–3 times per month, in order to review all of their human research protocols. Some institutions have additional oversight processes, for example, a separate committee may be in charge of reviewing the budget of each protocol, mainly to ensure that research costs and hospital treatment costs are allocated appropriately. There may be a central Office of Research Integrity that reviews the details of compliance with confidentiality issues (research projects require that information be deidentified, that is, that the name of the subject remains confidential and is not revealed in the process of the study, and that all information collected from the subject is linked to a coded number), potential conflicts of interest (whether an investigator may be receiving pay or have an interest in a company funding a drug trial), and the use of honest and verifiable methods in proposing, performing, and evaluating research.

At some institutions, this process is sequential such that the applicant may have to run the gauntlet of each of three separate reviews before being granted approval for their research project. In practice, each committee generally insists on reviewing the scientific validity of the project, regardless of the limitations of their mandates, be it budget, safety or conflicts of interest. This represents triple jeopardy to young investigators. In addition, the demands placed on the applicant can be multiplied. For example, a young investigator who, after reading many pages of posted "operating procedures" for each committee, is finally ready to submit a protocol. The integrity or oversight committee doing the review may have questions regarding the potential conflicts, confidentiality, and/or specific aims and experimental design. The budget oversight committee may have questions on the budget, methods, and consent forms. The IRB may also have questions related to several portions of the protocol. While each committee believes it is executing their charge dutifully and requests responses to increase their score by "only" 5 or 10 points, the investigator is faced with having to draft 15–30 responses. This is another case of triple jeopardy. Moreover, changes to a protocol at the second or third levels of review may require that the protocol be kicked back up the line and having to undergo another lengthy re-review process. In many cases, young investigators may need to resubmit their protocols several times. A successful clinician scientist with little time to spare could easily decide that such a process is simply not worth the effort.

What if the investigator believes that one or more of these reviews are arbitrary? This is perhaps the most discouraging prospect for a young scientist with options. While the IRB and other committees are charged with guarding the safety of human subjects, this mandate can easily be taken to extremes. The fact is that human nature being what it is, membership in such committees makes some people overzealous and obstructionist, mainly due to ignorance. If you constitute a witch-hunt, you will find a witch. Again, as with any review committee, good expertise and reasonable accommodation should be the standard. Rather than rejecting version after version of a protocol, rather than tabling for a question or voting to disapprove and require a resubmission, these committees need to assume the attitude of a facilitator rather than an obstructionist. Helping the investigator succeed without risking the safety of human subjects requires discussing the protocol with the investigator before it ever comes to a vote. Those institutions that can constitute committees with solid expertise, attention to regulations, and a helpful attitude will succeed, whereas others will fail.

Most CTSAs have a research support individual or office in order to help investigators navigate the regulatory quagmire. Given the limited support CTSAs receive from NIH, the institution will probably need to supplement this process in order to enable their human research protocols. Regardless of the investment in research support, if the IRB or similar regulatory committees consider themselves gatekeepers rather than facilitators, the institution and the investigators will be slowed unnecessarily, regardless of the investment. IRB reviewers and auditors who concentrate on the safety issues and procedures used on human research subjects are to be commended, those who obstruct research by concentrating on pagination, alternative titles, language use, and minutiae need to honestly question their motives. It is unfortunate that, human nature being what it is, those given power over others usually apply it to excess for no reason whatsoever.

The mentoring process to be described in detail below includes the identification of a Mentor for each of the young clinician scientists being trained as independent investigators. These Mentors prove their worth even before the research has started by helping to guide the young investigator through these obstacles. A Mentor with experience in regulatory processes is an invaluable resource. In addition, it is ideal for any translational research program, center, or institute to create a position for a Director of Clinical Research who oversees all of the protocols in the center and ensures that (a) approvals are secured expeditiously, (b) the protocols are set up appropriately (to avoid mistakes that can cost time and result in stoppages), and (c) all of the regulatory requirements are being met, especially during the early days of the research.

Fragmented infrastructure

Many institutions have some or all of the requisite facilities at some location or other across the academic health center. However, most are located where those who developed each of them needed them. For example, a Core Facility for recording evoked responses can be located in a department like Psychiatry, but a Transcranial Magnetic Stimulation (TMS) facility may be located in Neurology or Physical Medicine and Rehabilitation. Performing studies on the use of TMS for the treatment of tinnitus would force an Otolaryngology faculty member to guide subjects to two other sites in order to perform the research. This particular problem was addressed with the design of the CTSA program. Institutions were required by the NIH to establish an "Institute" for clinical and translational research, which would house the relevant infrastructure. The idea was to centralize much of the infrastructure needed for a variety of translational research efforts. The closer such facilities are located to one another, the more likely the success of the gamut of research projects. The proximity of research support personnel to the Core Facility personnel and to the source of patients or research subjects, the more efficient the effort invested by the institution, the Mentors and the clinician scientists in accomplishing their goals. In general, institutional training sessions, while helpful, do not provide sufficient in-depth instruction. Mentors need to take on additional monitoring duties to ensure that young investigators unfamiliar with the details of these regulations can be proactive.

Lack of qualified investigators

This is perhaps the most costly of the blocks to translational research. There is no doubt that prior experience in research is essential to success as a clinician scientist. Just as undergraduate research experience is a decided advantage to succeeding in graduate school, so is medical school and residency research essential to facilitating a translational research career. Involvement in summer research during medical school, in research rotations during senior year, and, of course, earning a MD/PhD, are all extremely advantageous to negotiating a successful translational research career. Nevertheless, institutions need to create the conditions that allow a young clinical faculty member to succeed in research, and we will discuss these under the T2 blocks to translational research. Another question is how to identify those who will have fruitful research careers. Aside from prior experience in research, which is really indicative of a long-standing interest on the part of the individual, institutions are making greater investments in their MD/PhD programs, accepting and supporting more students. In addition, those academic health centers that grant a full year of research in their residency and fellowship programs are more likely to grow their own translational research faculty. And, of course, it is the individual who keeps asking about research opportunities, does the leg work in meeting investigators in his/her area of interest, and is persistent in wanting to break into a research program, who is most likely to gain support and establish a viable career. Of course, the answer to the lack of qualified investigators is to train a cadre of dedicated clinician scientists. This is best accomplished through mentoring and a career development program that will be discussed following our consideration of the main blocks to T2 research.

T2 BLOCKS

Career disincentives

Most institutions have separate lines for promotion, with a clinical faculty line and a research faculty track. These usually entail milestones, a major one being the acquisition of a research award, that need to be met within a certain period of time, usually 7 years "up or out." If grant funding is an essential requirement for promotion, the pressures mount. However, the enterprise of grant funding has become so competitive that it is now making some of these milestones impossible to reach. For example, 30 years ago, the average age of a basic or clinical scientist who was awarded a first grant was 38 years of age. The current age of a faculty member garnering their first NIH grant award is 44 years of age for both MD and PhD applicants. If the faculty member begins a career at, say, 30 years of age, he/she is statistically unlikely to make promotion within 8–10 years. Without considerable help from a well-supported and effective Career Development Program, virtually no clinical faculty will enter the research track. Another issue was the fact that, before the doubling of the NIH budget, about 25% of the applicants were first-time investigators.

This percentage decreased to 23%, and only recovered to the 25% level by 2007.

NIH has responded to these barriers by establishing a New Investigator Award program that secures funding at a lower score than established investigators. The success rate in 1998 for first-time investigators was always lower that that of previously funded investigators (25% vs. 28%), both decreased in parallel until 2007, when they were virtually the same at ~19%. That is, the rate of funding for new investigators has been equalized to match that of established investigators. This bodes well for young clinician scientists attempting to break into the grant-funding field.

Practice limitations

Current medical practice makes translational neuroscience difficult to undertake. The need to generate salaries and clinical income now force young faculty into difficult choices. However, many department Chairs realize that a number of clinical faculty choose to practice medicine at an academic health center because of the research opportunities. A small number of these will actively seek a translational research career, and they can be some of the brightest recruits to a department. That is, creating opportunities for translational research on the part of young clinical faculty is an excellent recruitment and retention tool. With the help of a well-designed Career Development Program, support for translational research projects, and access to the appropriate Core Facilities, young faculty can lead stimulating and productive careers. They are also more likely to stay in academic medicine.

High research costs

The costs of translational research are usually higher than those of basic research, requiring some times as much as twice the yearly investment in funding. Most of the costs attendant to research, usually 70–90% of the total cost, are in personnel costs. The existence of a well-supported and staffed set of translational Core Facilities alleviates the need to support individual projects at such a high level. However, the single most expensive item in the personnel category is usually the young faculty's salary. The department wants to recover the costs of allowing their worker to spend time in the laboratory and not in the clinic, forcing the requested amount higher and higher. In addition, there are usually base salary levels that are supplemented with incentives, allowing academic health center salaries to at least approach those in private practice. How can a department afford to allow a young faculty member to spend a portion of their time doing research? How much time is required for a faculty member to generate grant support to meet these salary levels?

The fact is that it is unlikely that translational research projects can reach levels of salary support comparable to those of a busy practice. The key is to value the recruitment and retention of research-oriented faculty, and invest in their research program, especially in those who can garner grants as well as clinical trial funding. NIH awards typically have a maximum allowed for the base salary being requested by clinical faculty on a grant application, currently set at $199,700. Therefore, a faculty salary of, for example, $250,000 will never be fully supported even if the application requests 100% of the faculty's salary. In practice, a first award for a faculty member usually is well regarded by review committees at 25–50% of the base salary. In general, most NIH programs require that the faculty spend at least 50% of their time in research. This level of commitment is thought to be minimal in order to become competitive for grant funding and for developing the skills necessary for a successful independent research career. That means that departments and institutions must subsidize clinician scientists with potential for extramural funding. Some centers allow awards to pay as much as 25% of the base salary, and the department is required to match the other 25% of the base, thus establishing a partnership between the center or institute and the department in the investment on that faculty member. The department also must absorb the difference between the base salary and the full salary with incentives added. This is sometimes a burden for most departments, especially those with fewer faculty members such as Neurosurgery and Neurology, compared to Pediatrics and Psychiatry.

Institutions that provide the release time, at least 50%, for at least some clinician scientists, which have consolidated translational research Core Facilities, and which can support research projects by the young faculty, will reap the benefits of a vibrant translational research enterprise, with a CTSA institute, multiple translational research awards, and multiple clinical trials. The income derived by an institution from the indirect costs of these awards will help offset their investment, but, most of all, recruit and retain the best and the brightest.

Mentoring—a necessary solution to T1 and T2 blocks

A major element in the success of a young clinician scientist is the identification of the appropriate Mentor. Matching up a Mentee with a Mentor is no simple matter. Aside from being interested in the same research area, there has to be a certain chemistry between them. Considering the amount of time that they will spend together, the more compatible in other ways they are, the better. Incompatibilities can lead to a major waste of time and considerable frustration on the part of both scientists. In many cases, similarities in culture and/or ethnicity have been surprising elements in creating cohesive, productive research teams. In some cases, teams are formed as a result of social interactions at center functions, lectures, and laboratory meetings. In most institutions, the role of Mentor is not re-warded. Some centers do provide support for the important, altruistic work of Mentors, although it is usually nominal. The support should carry with it clearly outlined expectations, including the submission of biannual mentoring self-assessment forms documenting such mentoring activities as availability, questioning, skill development, networking, and the like. These forms create a history that allows one to assess progress, predict success, and some times prevent problems. An added benefit of establishing a coordinated relationship is that the Mentor and Mentee will tend to collaborate on research projects in the future, increasing the likeli-hood of funding for both of them.

The key to mentoring is the development of a successful Career Devel-opment Program for clinician and other translational research scientists by adopting the philosophy that we should be Mentors, not Tormentors. The approach is more efficient and reproducible if carried out through formal facilitation within a structure and with accountability rather than with a natural or situational mentoring approach, that is, by using sched-uled meetings, progress monitoring, and self-assessment tools. From the outset, the center needs to monitor all of the Mentor–Mentee partnerships and also participate in individual and team mentoring of every promising investigator in the program. This requires an open door policy designed to inspire and instill optimism (despite downturns in the funding situa-tion or regulatory setbacks), being ready to listen and be receptive, and to build friendships and communities. The impact will result in (a) facilitating funding for investigators, (b) facilitating recruitment of excellent faculty, (c) providing stability to the research programs of various departments, (d) increasing collaborations, (e) identifying and developing leaders in translational neuroscience research, (f) enabling maximum performance, (g) providing information for making career decisions, and (h) minimizing anxiety and indecision. A number of elements in a Career Development Program have been found to increase the chances of success.

Self-assessment

As the number of investigators being mentored grows, relevant materi-als are essential to assist Mentors in their role. A list of these materials is included in the reference list [2–8], and these materials should be dissemi-nated to new Mentors. An easy-to-use self-assessment tool was developed by Joan Lakoski, PhD, in the Department of Pharmacology and Chem-ical Biology at the University of Pittsburgh [9]. A translational research center should perform the self-assessment at least every 6 months, if not more often, to track progress. The results can be used to help the institu-tion develop a policy for the support of mentoring activities and provide guidelines for best practices across the institution. At institutions with-out CTSA awards, mentoring and Career Development Programs can be developed using the CTSA model. If a CTSA is awarded, there will already be an existing process that parallels CTSA guidelines. Tracking of mentoring success at least every 6 months allows one to determine the impact of (a) current mentoring efforts, (b) the implementation of mentoring in collaborative research (seelater), and (c) the compliance with the performance guidelines described in the following text.

Mentoring for collaborative research

The realities of modern translational research include a requirement for interdisciplinary and multidisciplinary research. While we can mentor a number of promising scientists to become independent investigators, the fact is that addressing complex clinical questions, applications, and therapies requires teamwork. It is advisable to develop mentoring sessions that include multiple Mentors and Mentees primarily centered on multidisciplinary projects, but widening the impact by including multiple teams of investigators and Mentors. These collaborative research mentoring sessions should emphasize, on the one hand, how to *establish* fruitful collaborations (discuss the usual types of collaborations, samples of collaborative situations, types of agreements, NIH and other agency regulations regarding collaborative research), and, on the other hand, how to *design* fruitful collaborations (discuss the design of multidisciplinary research, minimizing barriers to collaborative research, identifying potentially successful or undesirable collaborations). Because of the specialization and sophistication of modern biomedical research, collaborations become necessary whenever investigators wish to take their research program in a new direction, or realize the practical benefits of joint endeavors. A successful translational research center or institute needs to facilitate this process.

Established Mentor Program

Most successful centers have had, by definition, great success in matching established Mentors with research background and expertise appropriate to their respective Mentees. The Mentors for the projects all need to have considerable mentoring and multidisciplinary research experience, and know how to coordinate teams of junior and early career, clinical and basic, scientists. The Mentoring Plan described in the following text provides instruction on conducting research responsibly, improving the Mentee's self-confidence, critiquing and supporting the Mentee's research, defining a clear research focus, assisting in defining and achieving career goals, socializing the Mentee into the profession, assisting in development of extensive collegial networks, advising how to balance work and personal life, teaching more efficient utilization of resources, and assisting in the development of future colleagues, in addition to practical aid in experimental design, data collection/analyses, and grant application preparation.

External Speaker Program

Translational research centers need to invite several nationally and internationally prominent speakers per year, each an expert (and potential advisor or reviewer) in the area of research of each individual project. The invited speaker should interact primarily with the host project investigators. Because these guests will have expertise directly in the area of research or technology of each project, specific comments and suggestions for making each Project competitive can be canvassed by the center in order to improve funding potential. Personally hosting each speaker allows the investigators to show their results, interpretations, and enthusiasm to authorities in their field.

Biostatistics and Experimental Design

This program helps the project investigators with experimental design in the proposed studies and in future applications. The center needs to provide individualized instruction and advice in order to optimize access by the investigators to the center statistician. Questions of power analysis, data analysis and statistical applications for ongoing research, publications and future grant applications, should all be addressed. Attendance at a yearly institutional experimental design workshop should be required for those who have not participated previously such as new junior investigators.

Grant writing and reviews

Many centers support the costs of grant writing through an Office of Grants and Scientific Publications in order to optimize style and organization. The department some times supplements this endeavor through its ongoing support of that office, as needed. In addition to a translational center's Grant Strategy Sessions, in which center members freely critique an application, grant review or manuscript, the investigators should be allowed to seek advance reviews of grant applications to be submitted. Internal (senior center investigators could review all applications and request reviews from other institutional faculty) and paid external authorities in the relevant field, who have had NIH Review Committee experience, can be asked to submit written evaluations of the proposal using NIH guidelines. The center could also review critiques of applications that are not funded, and could request recommendations from external authorities in order to improve chances of funding for the resubmission.

Mentoring Plan

The term "mentor" can be traced back to the *Odyssey* of Homer, *Mentor* was Odysseus' friend, who was entrusted with the education of Odysseus' son, Telemachus. The word has come to denote an experienced advisor, a person who imparts wisdom, a counselor, coach, guide, or tutor. We need to take mentoring very seriously because of the impact it will have on the future of science. Implicit in the Career Development Plan is the Mentoring Plan, which, in addition to those issues discussed in the preceding text, involves the choice of compatible Mentors and Mentees to facilitate academic development at the faculty level. The role of the Mentors is to meet with the junior investigators on a regular basis to help in designing and critiquing experiments that test hypotheses, serve as a sounding board to solidify new ideas from the young scientists, review all manuscripts and advise them on appropriate journals for publications, introduce them to leaders in their field at scientific meetings, advocate for the Mentees as speakers at scientific meetings, and reviewers of manuscripts and grant applications, work with them on grant applications, especially those that will result from work done under the auspice of the center, give advice regarding hiring of personnel, including postdoctoral fellows, work with the Mentees in hosting visiting scholars, act as a proponent within the institution on their behalf, advise them on balancing research with teaching and service responsibilities, provide advice on personnel management issues, discuss and evaluate options regarding career development, interact with the Mentee as a faculty colleague, assist and advise them in the preparation of visual aids and slides for seminars and meetings, provide input on the preparation of posters for presentation, and listen to oral presentations for seminars, meetings, and other lectures.

The relationship between Mentors and early career investigators who have already competed successfully for support is different. Their inclusion in a mentoring plan provides them the opportunity to develop a second area of research, especially of collaborative investigations. Their Mentors are experts in the areas of proposed research and interact with them as peers, colleagues, and collaborators. A viable translational research center should expect significant scientific involvement of the Mentors and their laboratories with the early career faculty, which may result in additional co-authored publications and possible inclusion of the Mentor in joint grant proposals.

A final element of a typical Career Development Program, but no less important, is the setting of performance milestones. Center support cannot carry an open-ended timeframe or pocketbook. Therefore, the young investigator must meet these milestones in order to maintain that support. These can be used as guidelines and include (a) every investigator *must* submit a grant application by the end of the second year of funding or before; (b) such applications *must* be submitted to the center Director 2 months before the deadline to allow internal and/or external reviews prior to submission; (c) if such an application is not submitted, the Director and the Internal Advisory Committee (IAC), made up mostly of department Chairs, will work with the investigator to determine the cause(s) and find solutions, and a timetable will be set up with the Office of Grants and Scientific Publications to ensure timely progress, to be monitored by the Director; (d) the Director and the IAC may decide that funding will be terminated; (e) if the External Advisory Committee and the funding agency or source also concur will a replacement investigator be sought through the issuance of a request for proposals; (f) if the application submitted is not funded, a resubmission by the end of the third year of funding will be *required*; and (g) if the application is funded, the investigator will be considered to have "graduated" from the program and will retain access to the Core Facilities, unless the funded grant is in an area different from that involving the funded research, in which case the obligations of the investigator will continue, requiring an additional application by the end of one additional year of funding in order to maintain funding.

In conclusion, numerous obstacles impede translational research on multiple levels and from multiple angles, including recruiting enough participants, regulatory issues, lack of funding, fragmented infrastructure, career disincentives, and a lack of qualified investigators. Forging a strong partnership between Mentor and Mentee investigators and the development of a sound Career Development Plan for investigators supply young investigators with resources to aid in navigating through and overcoming these obstacles. European institutions are lagging in the implementation of such programs; however, a nonprofit European Mentoring and Coaching Council has been established with chapters in most European Union (EU) countries, and they are scheduling annual meetings starting in 2011. The focus is voluntary and community, professional training and development, counseling at work, life coaching, and academic psychology sectors. Therefore, the kind of focused program outlined here has a long way to go before it is implemented in the EU.

REFERENCES

1. The Belmont Report. (1979) Ethical Principles for the Protection of Human Subjects of Research. Department of Health, Education, and Welfare, National Commission for the Protection of Human Subjects of Biomedical and Behavioral Research. http://science.education.nih.gov/supplements/nih9/bioethics/guide/teacher/Mod5_Belmont.pdf.
2. DeLong TJ, Gabarro JJ, Lees RJ. (2008) Why mentoring matters in a hypercompetitive world: today's professional service firms are so busy making money that they've lost the art of making talent. Harvard Bus Rev 84, 115–121.
3. Detsky AS, Baerocher MO. (2007) Academic mentoring—how to give it and how to get it. JAMA 297, 2134–2136.
4. Jackson VA, Palepu A, Szlacha L, Caswell C, Carr PL, Inui T. (2003) Having the right chemistry: a qualitative study of mentoring in academic medicine. Acad Med 78, 328–334.

5. Lakoski JM. (2004) On being a savvy mentor and mentee: ethical responsibilities in a mentoring relationship. Endoc News 29, 15–17.

6. Leboy P. (2008) Fixing the leaky pipeline: why aren't there many women in the top spots in academia? The Scientist.http://www.the-scientist.com/2008/01/1/167/1/.

7. Lee A, Dennis C, Campbell P. (2007) Nature's Guide for mentors: having a good mentor early in your career can mean the difference between success and failure in any field. Nature Pub Group 447, 791–797.

8. Palepu A, Friedman RH, Barnett RC, Carr PL, Ash AS, Szlacha L, Moskowitz MA. (1998) Junior faculty members' mentoring relationships and their professional development in US medical schools. Acad Med 73, 318–323.

9. Keyser DL, Lakoski JM, Lara-Cinisomo S, Schultz DJ, Williams VL, Zellers DF, Pincus HA. (2008) Advancing institutional efforts to support research mentorship: a conceptual framework and self-assessment tool. Acad Med 83, 217–225.

3 Core Facilities for Translational Neuroscience

Edgar Garcia-Rill

Most institutions have an assortment of Core Facilities including Bioinformatics, Proteomic, Molecular, Cell Biology, Imaging, and similar dedicated agglomerations of sophisticated equipment. All of these are essential to running a vibrant research enterprise. However, while many clinician scientists are trained in one or more of these technologies, many more are not, and they depend on Core Facility personnel to carry out their research needs. Moreover, research aimed at molecular and cellular studies is beyond the time and effort that can be dedicated by unfunded, nascent clinician researchers. Thus, more often than not, the clinician scientist is more involved in securing samples or tissue for others to process. This is hardly conducive to helping establish a productive, independent research career. Therefore, the design of Core Facilities for translational neuroscience needs to accommodate the time constraints and the lack of high-end basic research experience.

The study of brain anatomy can be carried out with computer-assisted X-ray tomography (CT) and magnetic resonance imaging (MRI). These techniques provide high-resolution images of brain structure that are static, but they do not provide information regarding how the anatomy relates to brain function. While imaging brain structure is very desirable when considering developmental alterations, trauma, stroke, tumors, and other disorders in a research environment, the lack of prelesion or predisease imaging makes it less likely that definitive structural changes can be considered "causal." Moreover, many imaging studies do not reflect the actual nature of brain functioning that operates through the activation of multiple circuits working together simultaneously—not as isolated components operating independently. Therefore, these studies represent the subtraction of "control" or baseline activity in multiple brain systems from the postmanipulation or task demanded in a "test" condition, which may activate the same set of brain systems. While these provide interesting information,

Translational Neuroscience: A Guide to a Successful Program, First Edition. Edited by Edgar Garcia-Rill.
© 2012 John Wiley & Sons, Inc. Published 2012 by John Wiley & Sons, Inc.

the fact that the brain works through activation of multiple circuits simultaneously makes the subtraction of many events that occurred during both "control" and "test" seem rather artificial. By providing a result showing a single region resulting from this subtraction, these studies place undue emphasis on very specific regions "responsible" for a disease or disorder. Such differences could simply represent a difference in the functioning of a complex circuit that may or may not be causal to the symptoms observed. In addition, the higher and higher resolution of static images is coming at greater and greater imaging costs. The cost-benefit ratio of more and more detailed visualization will ultimately become too costly.

Given the constraints of static imaging in terms of its inability to determine causation of symptoms associated with brain functioning as well as its growing costs, it is important to consider other imaging methods to be used in translational research. Functional imaging is one such method, unlike static imaging, that focuses on identifying physiological activities such as metabolism, blood flow, chemical composition, or absorption within a certain tissue or organ. This type of imaging falls into two categories, hemodynamic/metabolic mapping and electromagnetic imaging methods, and they differ in terms of their spatial and temporal resolution.

In the first case, the coupling of increased neuronal electrical activity with local oxygen consumption, including increased blood flow, is used to indirectly identify anatomical regions involved in brain function. These include positron emission tomography (PET), which has a spatial resolution ~1 cm, and functional MRI (fMRI), which has a higher resolution ~1 mm. While these methods are valuable for identifying brain regions involved in brain function, they are limited by the rate of the metabolic event such as blood flow or oxygen consumption, so that their temporal resolution is ~1 second at best.

In the second case, electromagnetic techniques are able to directly measure ongoing brain activity in real time. Electrical events in single neurons occur in the 1–100-millisecond range. Thus, methods with temporal resolution ~1 second are too slow to study the rapid and complex brain dynamics involved in sensory perception, movement initiation, and cognitive processing. Two such noninvasive methods include electroencephalography (EEG) and magnetoencephalography (MEG). EEG measures electrical potential differences on the scalp, while MEG measures magnetic fields associated with current flow. Both methods have a temporal resolution ~1 millisecond and both measure synchronized brain activity. Chapter 6 will include a discussion of the uses of MEG. The remainder of this chapter will be devoted to other less expensive methods that allow multiple users to gather solid preliminary data useful for applying for funding and employing sophisticated methodologies targeting specific pathological processes.

Those institutional imaging facilities that have considerable time allotted for research are more likely to generate new funding for these investigators. However, part of the problem in terms of funding is that (a) the clinical demands almost require dedicated research machines and (b) this has become a very competitive field, making it difficult for neophytes to break into the funding cycles. Therefore, using alternative, cost-effective measures that produce reliable and valid quantitative measures of brain functioning is important.

DESIGNING TRANSLATIONAL NEUROSCIENCE CORE FACILITIES

Electrophysiology

How can you provide the infrastructure at a reasonable cost to accommodate the variety of possible translational neuroscience research opportunities? The answer is that it is unlikely, but there are methods and measures that are less expensive and can provide preliminary evidence for localizing the region or the process of interest in brain function. A variety of neurological and psychiatric disorders share disturbances in common processes and regions of the brain. For example, most neurological and psychiatric disorders are marked by dysregulation of sleep-wake, arousal, and attentional processing. These processes are localized to the brainstem, thalamus, and cortex. The simplest quantitative technique to use in measuring changes in state, sleep dysregulation, and the like is EGG. Although it has been around for ~75 years, it still provides solid diagnostic and reproducible measures in these processes. EEG studies in the clinical arena are used for the detection and diagnosis of sleep disorders. Because of its inability to provide punctiform localizability of events, the EEG does not afford sufficient physiological accuracy for, for example, surgical interventions. However, the fact is that EEG recordings show that we use many, many regions of the brain while simply "at rest," never mind when performing a complex task.

The EEG tells us about sleep and waking by recording the electrical activity of the brain. The EEG manifests high-frequency activity (detected as low-amplitude waveforms of many frequencies, usually cycling at 10–80 Hz or 10–80 cycles per second) during waking. The more alert and the more attention we pay to events or tasks, the higher the frequency of activation. It is thought that such activity represents the fact that very many cells are being modulated by graded membrane potentials and firing at different times in different, higher frequency patterns. Gamma band activity, which can be anywhere from 30 to 90 cycles per second, or Hz, is a sign of attention or sustained attention, and is thought to participate in such complex processes as learning and memory. This activity does not occur everywhere, being limited to cortical areas that may be activated individually or in sequence, exhibiting pockets of higher activation. As we become less active and eliminate visual input by closing our eyes, alpha band activity

~10 Hz becomes the predominant rhythm, especially over the occipital region. Alpha band can be thought of as the transition from waking to sleeping. If the oscillations slow down, it is thought that it is because more neurons become synchronized at lower frequencies and that more and more cells manifest graded potentials and action potentials at lower frequencies, thereby producing high-amplitude waveforms at low frequencies (<10 Hz) in the EEG characteristic of sleep. That is, "slow-wave" sleep is characterized by lower frequency activity that becomes progressively slower (from ~4–8 Hz called theta to ~1–4 Hz delta) with deeper and deeper sleep. If very large ensembles of cells are synchronized at very low frequencies, this essentially becomes an epileptic seizure. Every 90 minutes during slow-wave sleep, we manifest rapid eye movement (REM) sleep, in which, paradoxically, the EEG becomes activated and looks exactly like that during waking, that is, there is high-frequency, low-amplitude activity like in waking. However, during REM sleep, we undergo loss of muscle control called "atonia," basically so that we do not act out our dreams. Some investigators believe that memory consolidation can occur during REM sleep. In summary, the brain functions in a continuum and 10 Hz is the transition between sleep and waking, with lower frequencies being less conducive to such functions as learning and memory (and why we do not remember anything during epileptic seizures), and more complex functions better correlated with higher and higher frequencies of EEG activity.

An adjunct to the EEG is evoked potential recording studies. These involve stimulation of a sensory modality and averaging responses from brain regions, mainly primary sensory cortical areas (visual area for visual stimuli, auditory area for auditory stimuli, and so on). Brain responses that are time locked to an event of interest, such as a stimulus, will add while all other responses will cancel due to the nature of signal averaging. That is, if cortical cells respond to a stimulus with the same temporal response pattern, averaging will recover the response embedded in multiple trials with higher signal-to-noise ratio than that manifested on any single trial. These averages are assumed to be clearer estimates of evoked responses, and changes in amplitude, latency, and so on can be compared across subjects and experimental and pathological conditions. Unfortunately, during the development of this technique, someone noticed that following stimulation of each sensory modality only small regions of the brain were activated, and, as a group, covered only a small portion of the cortex. The erroneous impression was created that "we use only 10% of our brains" as a result of the kinds of studies that showed that only some of the cortical mantle was activated by stimulation of the primary afferent systems. Of course, this ignored the activation of many pathways that are not synchronized to the sensory stimulus and are averaged out. Needless to say, the more complex the task, the more brain regions that are activated. In fact, it is thought that evoked responses really represent a stimulus-induced resetting of ongoing neuronal oscillations seen in the EEG. Evoked potential research can provide more specific information than the EEG, and this technique tells us a lot about the brain.

Interestingly, evoked potentials elicited by activation of primary sensory pathways are only slightly affected by sleep–wake state. For example, a flash of light produces an evoked response over the occipital cortex whether it is delivered during waking or sleep, although the response is of somewhat lower amplitude during sleep. Similarly, auditory, somatosensory, and even olfactory stimuli are only mildly modulated by sleep–wake state. There is one evoked response that is sleep state-dependent is the P50 (P stands for positive and 50 stands for a 50-millisecond latency) midlatency auditory evoked potential. While the primary auditory cortex responds at ~25 milliseconds to an auditory stimulus, reflecting activation of the primary auditory pathways, the later arriving P50 potential is thought to reflect activation of arousal systems. That is, a click stimulus or a finger snap induces two responses, one through the auditory pathway that is thought to represent the "content" of auditory experience and one through the arousal pathways that is thought to represent the "context" of sensory experience. One is "what is it?", while the other is "wake up, something is happening!". The coincidence between these events at the level of the cortex is thought to represent one mechanism behind conscious experience [1].

PREATTENTIONAL MEASURE—THE P50 POTENTIAL

In order to measure the P50 potential, subjects are seated on a recliner in a well lit, sound attenuating, shielded room easily observed by the experimenter. Gold-plated surface electrodes are applied to the head with water soluble conducting paste, similarly to those used for EEG recordings. The signals are amplified and filtered to allow those waveforms within the frequency response range being studied, that is, if slow potentials are being recorded, the amplifiers use long time constants, if faster waveforms are being acquired, the time constants of the amplifiers are shorter. The P50 potential is recorded at the vertex (Cz) referenced to linked mastoids or other reference. Eye movements (EOG) are detected using diagonally placed canthal electrodes, while jaw movements (EMG) are detected using a lead over the temporalis muscle referred to the chin, both of which can provide artifacts to P50 potential recordings so that they are either averaged out or trials with excessive contamination are discarded. Prior to the recording, earphones are placed on each subject and the hearing threshold for each ear determined (usually ~25–35 dB, otherwise hearing loss is suspected). The test stimulus is usually a rarefaction click of 0.1-millisecond duration set at least 50 dB above hearing threshold, usually 85–103 dB. Testing sessions of 4–5 minutes in duration consist of paired click stimuli at a 250-, 500-, or 1000-millisecond interstimulus intervals (ISIs). Pairs of clicks are delivered once every 5 seconds (previous studies have shown that stimulation at faster frequencies can lead to a decrement in the P50 potential amplitude) until 64 pairs of evoked potentials are acquired, averaged, and stored by the computer. The use of three different ISIs allows one to develop a "recovery curve," basically a measure of the time it takes for the second stimulus to elicit a full-amplitude response, giving a measure of habituation to repetitive stimulation as the ISI is shortened. If the response to the second stimulus of a pair is higher than normal, then it can be said that the subject had impaired habituation to repetitive stimulation, or a deficit in sensory gating. Sensory gating is the property of the CNS critical to filtering unwanted information, making us better ready to respond to novel stimuli. Sensory gating deficits are characteristic of a number of psychiatric disorders.

A number of studies have established the characteristics of the P50 potential (it is sleep state-dependent, being present during waking and REM sleep, that is, during states of high-frequency activation; it undergoes rapid habituation, suggestive of a reticular rather than primary pathway waveform; and it is blocked by nonsoporific doses of the cholinergic antagonist scopolamine, suggesting it is modulated by cholinergic cells, those that use acetylcholine as a neurotransmitter), in contrast to the robust nature of the primary auditory cortex generated by the primary auditory cortex [present during all sleep–wake states, failed to habituate at high frequencies of stimulation and was unaffected by scopolamine]. Work on animal equivalents of the P50 potential lends support to the probable brainstem source of this waveform, suggestive of a reticular activating system (RAS) source, specifically, the pedunculopontine nucleus (PPN) (see Chapter 4, Section "TMS investigations in rodents"). The amplitude of the P50 potential is thus thought to be a measure of preattentional, brainstem-thalamus processing. The P50 potential also has been shown to exhibit characteristic abnormalities, especially in habituation, a component of *sensory gating*, in various psychiatric and neurological disorders, all of which are marked, and even presaged, by sleep disorders. As mentioned above, a measure of sensory gating can be derived from the use of paired stimuli to test the level of habituation in the system being studied. Important seminal studies using the P50 potential in pathological conditions revealed that schizophrenic patients did not inhibit the response to the second click stimulus under conditions in which normal subjects do show such reduced responsiveness, that is, there was a decrease in sensory gating. Schizophrenic patients show such sleep-related symptoms as reduced slow-wave sleep, reduced REM sleep latency, exaggerated startle response, and hallucinations.

The presence of decreased sensory gating of the P50 potential using a paired stimulus paradigm has been reported in another disorder marked by abnormalities of arousal and excitability, posttraumatic stress disorder (PTSD) in both male combat veterans and female rape victims. PTSD is also marked by such sleep–wake state-related abnormalities, as increased REM sleep drive hyperarousal, hallucinations, and exaggerated startle response. A similar decrease in sensory gating of the P50 potential was observed in patients in the late stages of Parkinson's disease (PD), suggesting that a sensory gating deficit can be present in these subjects. PD is characterized by a variety of symptoms that include resting tremor, rigidity, postural and gait abnormalities, bradykinesia, and freezing episodes. However, a majority of untreated PD patients show sleep disturbances including "light fragmented sleep," reductions in slow-wave sleep and frequent nocturnal arousals. Following treatment with levodopa, REM sleep appears to be suppressed. Interestingly, the decrease in habituation of the P50 potential was normalized in PD patients following bilateral pallidotomy for the relief of symptoms of the disease. These studies were the first to suggest that mesopontine cholinergic neurons of the RAS are *upregulated* in PD, and the normalization of P50 potential sensory gating following pallidotomy, a surgical procedure to eliminate a portion of a nucleus called the globus pallidus, was suggested to induce a reinhibition of PPN cells. The P50 potential also appears to undergo changes in *amplitude* as a result of other pathological states, being reduced in amplitude in patients with Alzheimer's disease (AD), autism, and narcolepsy, which is characterized by daytime somnolence, cataplexy, sleep paralysis and hypnagogic hallucinations. In general, then, the P50 potential is upregulated (increased amplitude and/or decreased sensory gating) in disorders that are marked by upregulation of RAS output and downregulated in disorders marked by decreased RAS output. Therefore, the amplitude of the P50 potential can be considered a measure of level of arousal, while its habituation using a paired stimulus paradigm can be considered a measure of sensory gating [2].

This makes the P50 potential, both its amplitude and its habituation, ideal for determining the presence of dysregulation of arousal and preattentional processes. Preattentional processes are essential for attentional processes, which are essential for learning and memory. That is, by determining if a patient with a specific disorder has preattentional problems, we can speculate that higher processes, such as attention and learning and memory, will also be disturbed. There are simple ways to assess attentional processes.

ATTENTIONAL MEASURES—PSYCHOMOTOR VIGILANCE

Simple attention is critical for a number of processes, including selective or sustained attention, learning, and memory. The prototypical test of attention is reaction time (RT), or the ability to reply promptly to a stimulus, and it is thought to be mediated by thalamocortical processes. The psychomotor vigilance task (PVT) is a test of behavioral alertness and involves a simple (not choice) RT test designed to evaluate the ability to sustain attention and respond in a timely manner to salient signals [3]. The PVT was designed to be simple to perform, to be free of a learning curve or influence from acquired skills (aptitude, education), and to be highly sensitive to an attentional process that is fundamental to normal behavioral awareness. The PVT consists of responding to a 90 dB tone of 1000-Hz frequency by pressing a response button as soon as the stimulus appears, which stops the stimulus counter and displays the RT in milliseconds for 1 second. The ISI varies from 2 to 10 seconds, and the task typically lasts 10 minutes (which yields 80 RTs per trial). The subject is instructed to press the button as soon as each stimulus appears, in order to keep the RT as low as possible, but not to press the button too soon (which yields a false start—FS warning on the display). Special software will be used to extract multiple performance parameters from each PVT trial: (1) *frequency of lapses*, which refer to the number of times the subject fails to respond to the signal or fails to respond in a timely manner; (2) *duration of lapse domain*, which refers to shifts in lapse duration calculated from the slowest 10% RTs, a measure that reflects vigilance response slowing; (3) *optimum response times*, which are the average of the fastest 10% RTs per trial, and reflect the very best performance an operator is capable of producing; (4) *fatigability function*, which refers to the vigilance decrement function or the extent to which subjects maintained performance across time on task; (5) *false response frequency*, which refers to the number of responses that were initiated when no stimulus was present; and (6) the visual analog rating (selected by the investigator) made by the subject at the end of the PVT trial. These PVT performance variables can be compared to values from the same subjects at different times, to known populations of control or pathological subjects, and so on. The compact, portable nature of the PVT, its sensitivity as a task, and its documented sensitivity to the fundamental neurobehavioral function of sustained attention make it ideal for tracking test conditions, disease progression, and/or therapeutic efficacy.

Now that we can assess preattentional and attentional systems are there relatively simple and economical ways of measuring higher cortical function?

FRONTAL LOBE BLOOD FLOW MEASURES

Near infrared spectroscopy (NIRS) measurement is made by passing harmless near infrared light through the patient's forehead and into the brain. In the near infrared band, light scatters easily through tissues. The depth of the light signal is related to the distance between the light source and the photo detectors. Since the majority of blood in the region of the brain is venous blood, changes in values are influenced by the critical balance between arterial oxygen delivery and cerebral consumption. Imbalances are identified by changes in regional oxygen saturation, rSO_2. These machines are oximeters that use a Class 1 laser, which has a nominal output of 0.5 milliwatts (mW). A Class 2 laser has a nominal output of 1.2 mW. Class 1 and Class 2 lasers are used in stores for scanning bar codes. The new laser pointers used in the classroom are more powerful and are classified as Class 3a lasers. Even the more powerful Class lasers produce no thermal effects and the only damage that could result is to the retina but only after staring directly into the beam for an extended period. The near infrared frequency of light used is in the range used for remote controllers for TVs and DVD players. Most DVD players use a Class 1 laser to "read" the disk. That is, Class 1 lasers are now ubiquitous and are harmless.

The clinical tissue oxygenation monitors are used to measure changes in hemoglobin concentration and the redox state of cytochrome oxidase, as well as the ratio of oxygenated to total tissue hemoglobin. In NIRS, the slope of light attenuation versus distance is measured at a distant point from the light input, from which the ratio is calculated using light diffusion theory. Laser diodes are used as the light source. A high gain, low-noise amplifier is used in the detector, enabling a large emitter-detector separation of ~5 cm. Placement of electrodes on the forehead can measure relative, not absolute, frontal lobe blood flow changes, and using two electrodes, comparisons between right and left frontal blood flows can be made. These monitors are used clinically in rehabilitation/orthopedic settings, in neonatal ICU (continuous brain blood flow measured over the fontanelle), and to assess hypofrontality in mood disorders during the performance of cognitive tasks [4].

Taking into consideration these measures, such a Human Electrophysiology Core Facility, thus provides a preattentional measure of brainstem-thalamus processes, an attentional measure of thalamocortical processes, and a measure of frontal lobe blood flow that can speak to higher functions. By providing such screening over a matter of 1 hour, a large number of subjects can be assessed and conclusions about the level of the brain system involved can be advanced. For example, changes in frontal lobe blood flow in the absence of other changes suggest that PET scans of frontal glucose metabolism would be very useful and provide a fruitful direction for research. Disturbances in PVT scores in the absence of P50 potential amplitude changes suggest that thalamocortical systems are involved, but brainstem mechanisms are fairly intact. Disturbances in the habituation of the P50 potential, but not its amplitude, can also speak to a lack of frontal lobe function that indicates reduced outflow or lack of inhibition of repetitive stimuli. Of course, significant changes in the amplitude of the P50 potential are indicative of hyperarousal if amplitude is increased, or hypoarousal if amplitude is decreased, compared with normal levels. This array of techniques allows any investigator to study all of these processes in virtually any brain disorder, and to compare these measures with those taken after interventions, whether surgical, pharmacological, or behavioral. These indices can be used to track disease progression as well as to monitor therapeutic efficacy easily and at low cost.

We have developed Animal Electrophysiology, Molecular and Cell Biology, Behavioral, Transcranial Magnetic Stimulation (TMS), Telemedicine, and Cellular Imaging Cores, as well as an Administrative Core. Other chapters in this book will describe the Electrophysiology (using parallel human and animal models to study comparative physiology), TMS (as a form of treatment for a number of disorders), and Telemedicine (an excellent example of community-based research) Cores in detail. While the Molecular and Cell Biology and Behavioral Cores are fairly standard, an unusual combination of pieces of equipment may be needed in the Cellular Imaging Core Facility well suited to undertake a number of translational research efforts, as will be discussed next.

Cellular Imaging

The presence of a confocal microscope is standard across most Image Analysis Core Facilities, and these usually include a morphometric software package allowing the user to perform quantitative analyses of cell number, cell structure, and three-dimensional reconstruction of cells and nuclei. Another imaging approach is the use of voltage-sensitive dyes or calcium imaging dyes. These fluorescent labels change, as their names imply, with membrane voltage or calcium concentration. Such studies are typically done on slices of brain tissue, which could be from animal sources or from surgical resections from surgery of epileptic tissue or tumors. For example, slices containing the PPN, which generates the P50 potential in humans, can be used to study the cellular properties of a region involved in this waveform in truly translational studies. In order to facilitate a number of different approaches, multiple camera systems may be required. Whether measuring synaptic vesicle recycling or looking at dose–response studies within a brain region, three camera parameters define the scope and quality of image data collection for translational neuroscience: sensitivity, speed, and resolution.

Sensitivity

For the majority of imaging applications commonly encountered in neuronal studies, the sample used will emit very low levels of light. Regardless of experimental setup and tissue of interest, a central dogma for all pharmaceutical research is to determine the minimal effective dose for the drug under investigation. Additionally, large concentrations of fluorescent dyes and other labels can have unexpected effects on cellular behavior and biomolecular reactions. Such imaging markers are consequently used very conservatively. In general, minimal use of both pharmaceuticals and labeling reagents makes sense. However, this also provides a significant challenge when attempting to image and document the effects of low-concentration drugs. Small drug dosages can produce minute effects on cellular mechanisms, which are monitored with even smaller concentrations of imaging markers, and results in an extremely low-light flux from the sample and places significant demands on the camera's performance. These dim signals, due in part to minimal use of dye labels and dosage size, are also a result of the high-speed imaging requirements. High frame rates require short integration times that vastly limit the amount of light captured with each exposure of the sensor. These three factors create a situation where the sample image is nearly indistinguishable from the noise unless an imaging device with incredibly low-noise, high-quantum efficiency (QE), and a large area of collection (pixel area) is used.

For these extreme low-light applications, highly sensitive, back-illuminated electron multiplying charge-coupled device (EMCCD) cameras are generally recommended. Through multiplying the signal electrons by factors of 1000 or more before readout, the electron multiplying capabilities of EMCCDs reduces effective read noise (the predominant source of noise when detecting low levels of light) below 0.5 electrons. This low noise, in combination with peak QEs (the fraction of photons of light converted into signal electrons) greater than 92%, makes back-illuminated EMCCD cameras the most sensitive cameras for scientific imaging. Additionally, EMCCD sensors are often comprised of large pixels, as a larger area per pixel directly correlates to a larger amount of light each pixel will capture and detect. While this results in a decrease in spatial resolution, it is more important in low-light applications that the signal is detected and quantitatively measured.

When sensitivity is the dominant parameter of interest, it is advisable to use cameras like either the Evolve 128 or the Evolve 512 (Photometrics Inc., AZ). As a general workhorse camera for many translational neuroscience applications, the Evolve 512 EMCCD camera provides ultimate sensitivity with significant field of view and high speed. Taking advantage of back-illuminated sensitivity (92% peak QE) and electron multiplying technology, it can distinguish signals well below the detection limit of standard interline CCDs without the need for exposure times exceeding 1 second. The Evolve 512 employs a back-illuminated, 512×512 EMCCD sensor with 16-μm pixels. At full frame, this camera is capable of streaming at 31 frames per second, which provides excellent temporal resolution at a large field of view. For experiments that require an even higher temporal resolution, the smaller format Evolve 128 (128×128 EMCCD sensor) is recommended.

Speed

Biochemical reactions in tissue and neuronal activities are often nearly instantaneous events that can easily be missed by slow speed cameras. If a reaction only spans 250 milliseconds, a camera running at 15 frames per second at most captures 3–4 frames of meaningful data. With this limited amount of information, it is difficult to make conclusions and accurately describe the reaction taking place. For this reason, it is imperative that the researchers use a camera with high frames rates. More data points result in a greater detail of information and a better understanding of the reaction. The vast majority of neuronal research initiatives involve tracking changes in signal intensity over time to determine if the introduction of a pharmaceutical induces some degree of change. A common example of this scenario would be dose–response studies. Resolving finite details within the sample are less important than quantitatively measuring a statistically significant change for this type of experiment, meaning that speed and sensitivity take precedence over resolution.

Maximum frame rates can be achieved by small format CCD cameras with limited resolution. However, speed alone is not sufficient for most neuronal studies, as the levels of light emitted from the samples are typically below the detection limits for standard interline CCDs at the necessarily ultrafast exposures. As a result, the ideal camera for high-speed, low-light imaging applications is a small array back-illuminated EMCCD camera. The Evolve 128 camera from Photometrics, which contains a 128×128, 24-μm pixel, back-illuminated EMCCD sensor, can run at a full frame rate of 530 frames per second. This extreme frame rate enables exceptional temporal resolution. Where the 15 frames per second camera could only capture 3 data points, this camera would capture 125 data points. Clocking at 530 frames per second puts incredible stress on camera electronics. As a result, a common problem encountered with EMCCD cameras running this fast is the stability of the camera bias (baseline) and EM gain. It is critical in scientific imaging that changes in image intensity result from effects within the sample itself and not from drift in the camera background and gain levels.

Resolution

Once dose–response and signal change have been documented over a time scale, localization and area studies are necessary to identify affected tissue areas and determine drug permeability. For these experiments, a large field of view and high resolution are the key camera parameters. The field of view is important for identifying affected areas in population response studies, and covering the same field of view with higher resolution enables easier resolution of finer details in the tissue sample. However, this increased resolution requires a tradeoff in sensitivity, as resolving smaller sample features requires smaller pixels, so that less light can be collected per pixel due to each pixel's smaller collection. While a compromise must be partially made in terms of sensitivity to provide higher resolution images for greater spatial information, this sensitivity can also be regained through the use of EMCCD cameras that are able to reduce the noise floor to below 0.5 electrons.

While the Evolve 512 provides high sensitivity and improved resolution over the Evolve 128, additional resolution to resolve finer features may be needed in some studies. The Evolve 512 provides a good balance of spatial resolution and field of view at high magnifications. However, a camera that uses an array of a larger number of smaller pixels would allow the ability to resolve smaller features at the same high magnifications or the ability to resolve similar size features with a larger field of view using somewhat smaller magnifications. Examples where higher resolution would be advantageous include the analysis of the distribution of pharmacological effects in large populations of cells, and the localization of drug binding and induced structural changes in organelles at the subcellular level. In neuronal studies requiring higher resolution, simply replacing a back-illuminated EMCCD camera such as the Evolve 512 with a high-resolution interline CCD camera will most likely not produce images with sufficient signal to be distinguished above the image noise. Again, this results from the low-light levels intrinsic to most neuronal and pharmacological experiments. As mentioned earlier, smaller pixels, as would be used in higher resolution cameras, reduce the area used by each pixel to collect light emitted from the sample, resulting in reduced sensitivity. Additionally, interline CCDs are typically front-illuminated, rather than back-illuminated, resulting in a somewhat lower QE (often around 65%) due to some light loss by the electronics on the front of the sensor and thus lower sensitivity. Finally, an interline CCD will have a typical read noise (the limiting noise factor in low-light imaging) of around 6 electrons, significantly higher than the <0.5 electron read noise of EMCCDs, for a further drop in sensitivity.

For these high-resolution experimental studies, in addition to the need for higher spatial resolution, the other requirements for neuroscience research still apply, namely, high speed with low noise and high sensitivity. High camera frame rates are still required to capture rapidly occurring biochemical reactions within the cell or short-lived neuronal events. With the high frame rates come short exposure times that afford little time for a camera to collect light and thus require high sensitivity either through high QE or low noise, such as the sub-electron read noise provided by electron multiplying gain in EMCCDs. In order to achieve the requirements for high-speed, low-light neuronal imaging with the addition high-resolution imaging for experiments where it is required, the Rolera EM-C^2 EMCCD camera is an excellent choice. It contains a front-Illuminated 8 µm 1004×1002 CCD array with a QE of around 65%. Although with front-illumination its QE is somewhat lower than the Evolve cameras, the EM-C^2 is still also an EMCCD, meaning that it can also achieve <0.5 electron read noise for the high-sensitivity capability with electron multiplication. The EM-C^2 EMCCD can also perform high-spatial resolution pharmaceutical studies with pixels half the size of the Evolve 512, meaning that at the same magnification it can resolve features half the size of what the Evolve 512 could. When performing population dose–response experiments where resolution is less critical and field of view is the key parameter, the EM-C^2 can take advantage of its large array size (approximately twice the number of pixels in height and width) by using a lower magnification to achieve similar spatial resolution, but with approximately twice the width and height of the field of view and around four times the captured sample area. Additionally, the EM-C^2 EMCCD camera achieves the high imaging speeds needed to reach the high-temporal resolution needed for most neuroscience applications through its maximum full frame rate of 34 frames per second and a >100 frame per second rate for region of interest single cell imaging.

Therefore, a full-service cellular imaging facility must be able to fulfill a wide array of requirements that optimize sensitivity, speed, and resolution. The investment in an array of cameras that have overlapping but functionally distinct features allow a Cellular Core Facility the capability of serving a wide array of translational neuroscience applications.

REFERENCES

1. Llinas R. (2001) I of the Vortex, from Neurons to Self. Cambridge, MA: The MIT Press.
2. Garcia-Rill E, Skinner RD. (2001) The sleep state-dependent P50 midlatency auditory evoked potential. In: Lee-Chiong TL, Carskadon MA, Sateia MJ, eds. Sleep Medicine. Philadelphia: Hanley & Belfus, pp. 697–704.
3. Dinges D, Powell A. (1985) Microcomputer analyses of performance on a portable, simple visual RT task during sustained operations. Behav Res Meth 17, 652–655.
4. Al-Rawi PG, Smielewski P, Kirkpatrick PJ. (2001) Evaluation of a near-infrared spectrometer (NIRO 300) for the detection of intracranial oxygenation changes in the adult head. Stroke 32, 2492–2500.

4 Translational Studies Using TMS

Mark Mennemeier, Christine Sheffer, Abdallah Hayar, and Roger Buchanan

OVERVIEW

Chapter 1 described translational research as both circular and bidirectional. Translational research is circular because it can begin at any point in the bench-to-bedside-to-community cycle. It is bidirectional because a discovery at one point in the cycle can prompt research in the following or previous stages. For example, a basic science discovery might prompt a clinical trial and/or a clinical discovery might prompt basic research concerning mechanisms of change. Making a clinical treatment available to the public, yet another stage of research translation, typically requires both basic research and clinical trials in order to gain Food and Drug Administration (FDA) approval. Each of the studies described in this chapter supports a common goal of making transcranial magnetic stimulation (TMS, a noninvasive form of brain stimulation) available to the public as a treatment; however, the studies themselves represent different applications and different stages of the translational research cycle. TMS is regarded by the FDA as an investigational device, and it was only recently granted limited approval for the treatment of depression [15]. Our studies using TMS to treat tinnitus (phantom sound perception) are specifically designed to translate clinical findings into general medical practice by laying the foundation for a large-scale trial that can gain FDA approval for this application. For example, our initial efforts to apply TMS for the treatment of tinnitus [1,2] prompted a laboratory study to develop a realistic placebo or sham TMS [3] technique that is described in Section "Development of a sham stimulation technique for humans." Similarly, we have conducted studies to improve the targeting of TMS, to define treatment responders, and to develop schedules of TMS delivery that will also be part of a larger clinical trial. These findings are described in Section "PET-guided TMS

Translational Neuroscience: A Guide to a Successful Program, First Edition. Edited by Edgar Garcia-Rill.
© 2012 John Wiley & Sons, Inc. Published 2012 by John Wiley & Sons, Inc.

studies of tinnitus perception." Studies described in Sections "TMS investigations of decision-making in tobacco addiction" and "TMS investigations in rodents" focus on tobacco addiction, and they are designed to discover mechanisms of change in TMS. In general, the clinical usefulness of TMS has outpaced knowledge of its neural mechanisms of action [4], and there is a great need for basic science studies of TMS [4]. Section "TMS investigations of decision-making in tobacco addiction" describes a study of TMS to alter cognition and behavior in persons who are tobacco dependent. This study examines whether and how TMS influences dopamine reward systems in smokers who are either satiated or withdrawn from nicotine. Section "TMS investigations in rodents" describes a parallel study of TMS effects in rodents exposed to nicotine that affords a greater opportunity to examine neural mechanisms of action. All of the studies described in this chapter will inform the design of clinical trials in human subjects that are necessary to translate TMS into clinical practice. We now turn to necessary background material on TMS.

INTRODUCTION

TMS induces stimulation of cortical neurons by creating a brief, focused magnetic field over the surface of the brain. Magnetic fields may be administered at frequencies ranging from 0.3 to 50 Hz or more, depending on limitations of the stimulator, and they can reach intensity levels of 2 T. Magnetic fields pass unimpeded through the scalp and skull and induce small electrical fields within the brain by creating transmembrane potentials [5]. The magnetic field induced by TMS is brief (microseconds) and declines rapidly with distance away from the coil [5,6]. Up to 3 cm of cortex may be stimulated directly beneath standard coils; however, deeper brain structures can also be affected via cortical–subcortical connections [7]. As such, TMS is noninvasive and can be administered at multiple cortical locations in human subjects with minimal discomfort. Magnetic fields beneath the coil also cause cutaneous scalp stimulation and muscle twitching and perhaps contraction of vessels in the brain. Scalp stimulation is primarily what a subject feels during TMS and it confounds attempts to disguise TMS in controlled placebo or sham stimulation conditions. When magnetic pulses are delivered repetitively and rhythmically, the process is called repetitive TMS (rTMS) and is commonly used in clinical applications to prolong the duration of the effect. The motor threshold (MT) of TMS typically refers to the minimal intensity of magnetic stimulation necessary to elicit a muscle contraction of the thumb or fingers of the contralateral hand when the motor cortex is stimulated. MT is used in most rTMS studies to tailor the intensity of stimulation given to an individual subject. It is the primary means of reporting TMS intensity, that is, as a percentage of the MT, and referencing intensity within and across subjects and studies.

The effect of TMS on local neuronal populations can be excitatory or inhibitory [8], and its duration can last seconds to weeks (or longer) depending on how TMS is delivered. Low-frequency stimulation of a single neuron produces long-lasting inhibition of cell–cell communications (long-term depression) [9,10], whereas high-frequency stimulation improves cell–cell communication (long-term potentiation) and produces excitatory effects [11–14]. The duration of TMS effects is influenced by stimulation parameters such as the intensity, frequency, and number of pulses delivered to a subject across one or more TMS sessions. In general, TMS effects are prolonged by applying stimulation repetitively, by increasing the number of pulses given per session, and by repeating treatment sessions over several days. Immediate effects of TMS are thought to result from direct excitation of inhibitory or excitatory neurons, whereas intermediate effects of TMS, occurring minutes after stimulation, may depend on changes in local pharmacology. Long-term effects that may last for days or months are not well understood at the present time. Notwithstanding our limited knowledge of mechanisms, several double-blind, randomized, sham-controlled trials have recently demonstrated that both high-frequency left prefrontal [15–17] and low-frequency right prefrontal TMS [15,18] have antidepressant effects, and the FDA has granted limited approval of rTMS for treating depression. In fact, the range of disorders in which TMS has been shown to have some clinical benefit is large, including (but not limited to) auditory hallucination in schizophrenia, posttraumatic stress disorder, drug craving, Parkinson's disease, dystonia, epilepsy, and various perceptual disorders such as tinnitus and certain pain syndromes [4]. Our center has focused on applying rTMS to treat tinnitus and to alter cognition and behavior in tobacco addiction. The following sections provide examples of the types of translational research studies being conducted that support our clinical applications.

DEVELOPMENT OF A SHAM STIMULATION TECHNIQUE FOR HUMANS

In order to conduct placebo-controlled clinical rTMS trials, there must be an appropriate sham or control condition that replicates the look, sound, and feel of active stimulation. Our laboratory developed and validated a new method of sham rTMS appropriate for a double-blind, placebo-controlled study [3]. The look and sound of active rTMS was replicated using a matched, air-cooled sham TMS coil that produces a biologically inactive magnetic field. The feel of rTMS is produced using large rubber electrodes placed over selected muscles beneath the stimulation coil (see Figure 4.1). These electrodes are in place for every TMS session but only during sham stimulation, is a small electrical current delivered to target

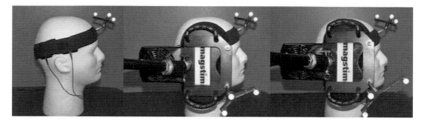

Figure 4.1   Active and sham stimulation. Large carbon rubber electrodes (left image) stimulate scalp muscles electrically during sham (right image) but not active (middle image) stimulation to replicate the feel of rTMS.

muscles, which is timed to coincide precisely with the clicking sounds made by the sham TMS coil. In this way, the muscle twitching associated with *verum* TMS is replicated by electrical stimulation during sham TMS. The sham technique was validated in back-to-back comparisons with active rTMS at 1 Hz. Subjects, naïve to rTMS and condition, were unable to accurately identify active from sham stimulation beyond a chance level of performance. However, we and others [19] found that naïve subjects are biased such that they more frequently (and incorrectly) identified the sham stimulation as active, stating that the electrical stimulation felt more focused than magnetic stimulation, and thus more closely fit their expectations of rTMS. In fact, nine of ten participants chose electrical stimulation as the active form of stimulation when asked to guess ($p < 0.05$) following back-to-back comparisons. Subjects who had previous experience with rTMS were more able than naïve subjects to correctly identify the sham and active stimulation conditions in back-to-back comparisons. As mentioned later, we find that, in treatment studies in which subjects receive weeklong courses of active or sham stimulation rather than back-to-back comparisons, they are not able to identify conditions beyond chance, and they are not biased to choose one type of stimulation as either active or sham.

Implications for translational applications

This method of providing a sham or control condition for rTMS closely mimics the look, sound, and feel of active stimulation. It is valid for use with parallel or crossover treatment designs. It can accommodate differences in scalp muscle recruitment, so it can be used at multiple treatment sites. Finally, we have now validated the technique for use with high- and low-frequency stimulation that is reported in Section "TMS investigations of decision-making in tobacco addiction."

PET-GUIDED TMS STUDIES OF TINNITUS PERCEPTION

Tinnitus refers to the perception of sound (i.e., ringing, hissing, or buzzing) in the absence of external stimulation. This disorder affects one in five adults in the United States and is disabling for as many as one in ten of sufferers [20]. There is no cure for tinnitus and no widely effective form of treatment at the present time. Medications are used to treat associated depression and anxiety but are not more effective for treating tinnitus than placebo. The proposed etiology of tinnitus has both peripheral and central components [1,2,21–25]. Sensory deafferentiation due to peripheral injury may incite tinnitus, but central components such as thalamocortical dysrhythmia and cortical reorganization appear to promote and maintain tinnitus [23,26]. Recent studies, several of which have been conducted in our laboratory, indicate that low-frequency rTMS delivered over the auditory cortex can reliably ameliorate tinnitus for approximately 50% of patients [1,25,27–29]. Other frequencies and sites of stimulation have also proven effective for tinnitus, but the majority of studies apply low-frequency stimulation to either the right or left temporal cortex [30]. One problem associated with rTMS treatment for tinnitus as well as other disorders is its short-lived effect. A course of rTMS involving daily sessions for 5–10 days may only provide relief for 1–2 weeks. In order to test the hypothesis that tinnitus is produced by asymmetric, excessive cortical activity in the temporal lobes, we used positron emission tomography (PET) imaging to target treatment sites in patients with tinnitus and to assess change in cerebral metabolism and blood flow after treatment [31]. We also aimed to determine whether the added precision of targeting the coil afforded by pretreatment PET imaging improved the percentage of persons who respond positively to rTMS treatment.

Methods

Twenty-one adults with moderate to severe tinnitus aged 28–75 years were enrolled in this sham-controlled, crossover study that used 1-Hz rTMS applied at an intensity of 110% of the MT and a rate of 1 Hz for 30 minutes (1800 pulses per session) every day for five consecutive days. Most subjects also had mild to moderate hearing loss and tinnitus severity, and none were depressed (see [31] for details). All subjects were diagnosed with idiopathic subjective tinnitus, and all were free of risk factors for TMS including prior significant head injury, medication that alters seizure threshold, and a first degree relative with a seizure disorder. Subjects were randomly assigned to receive five sessions of either active or sham treatment first, with 1 week intervening the sham and active treatment sessions. The sham stimulation technique was that described in Section "Development of a sham stimulation technique for humans."

PET scans were used to locate areas of increased neuronal activity in the temporal cortex and target rTMS delivery. However, one-third of subjects did not have significant temporal lobe PET asymmetries or had asymmetries located deep within the temporal or inferior lobe and not accessible to rTMS. Temporal lobe asymmetry identified by the PET scan was targeted when they were clear and accessible to rTMS (62% of subjects). When no

PET asymmetry was present, the posterior one-third of the superior temporal gyrus opposite the ear with the loudest tinnitus was targeted (33%). When tinnitus could not be lateralized and when no PET asymmetry was present, the same location in the left hemisphere was targeted (5%). Targeting the left temporal lobe is a standard approach in the literature [32]. On the basis of these criteria, the right temporal lobe was targeted for treatment in 62% of subjects and the left temporal lobe was targeted in 38%.

The primary outcome measures were the ear-specific visual analog ratings of tinnitus loudness (VARL) (0 = tinnitus absent; 100 = extremely or painfully loud tinnitus) assessed at baseline, before and after each day of treatment, and during the week following treatment, and differences in the PET scans before and after treatment. The dependent measure used in the analysis was change in the VARL from pre- to postactive and sham treatment, expressed as a percentage of the pretreatment score. We identified responders as those who achieve >33% reduction in the VARL in either ear following active treatment. PET analyses were performed using the NeuroQ™ Display and Analysis Program (Cardinal Health, Dublin, Ohio, Version 2.0). The primary region of interest (ROI) for data analysis was an area over the superior lateral temporal cortex of the right and left hemispheres where rTMS was applied. The effect of rTMS on the VARL for each ear was evaluated using a 2 (treatment type: sham or active) by 2 (side of rating: ipsilateral or contralateral to rTMS) by 2 (treatment order: active or sham first) mixed model, three-way analysis of variance (ANOVA).

Results

A significant three-way interaction between treatment type, side of rating, and treatment order (F (1, 18) = 6.10, $p < 0.03$) was observed for the VARL. An order effect (F (1, 18) = 6.77, $p < 0.02$) was observed such that when active treatment came first, a significant carryover effect was observed into the sham treatment week for the ear contralateral to treatment ($F = 11.5$, df = 18, 1, $p < 0.003$), that is, the VARL was decreased from baseline by 31% (SE = 8) at the end of the sham treatment week. A similar but marginal effect was observed for the ear ipsilateral to treatment ($p < 0.064$), which was decreased by 12% (SE = 9) from baseline. In contrast, when sham treatment came first, ratings of tinnitus loudness were not significantly different from pretreatment either for the ear contralateral or ipsilateral to rTMS. No detrimental effects of active or sham rTMS were observed on any tests, and there were no changes in hearing at the end of treatment. Neither the tinnitus severity index (TSI) nor the beck depression inventory (BDI) changed significantly from baseline as a result of either active or sham treatment.

To learn what stimulation site was associated with a positive response to rTMS, a subtraction procedure (MRIcron) was used that identifies ROIs common to subjects who respond positively to rTMS but not to those who

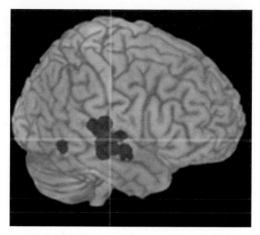

Figure 4.2   Region of interest plot. A circular "region of interest" denotes the location of each treatment site. A subtraction procedure (in MRICroN) revealed sites common to participants who responded (i.e., BA 22, designated by the crosshair) but not to nonresponders. (For color detail, please see the color plate section.)

failed to respond to rTMS. Positive responses to rTMS were associated with targeting treatment over secondary auditory cortex (Brodmann's area 22) (see Figure 4.2).

Analysis of the PET data at the primary treatment site revealed a significant interaction of treatment site and time (F (1, 12) $= 7.01$, $p < 0.05$) such that metabolic activity was decreased significantly beneath the stimulation coil after rTMS. Whereas this result is consistent with the expected effect of 1-Hz rTMS, similar significant findings were observed in control sites located over visual, parietal, and sensory motor cortices that were not predicted to change. Additionally, the effect of treatment response was not significant in any of the ANOVA models, and change in tinnitus loudness following active rTMS did not correlate significantly with change in PET activity at the site of TMS ($r = 0.33$ for the ipsilateral or $r = 0.27$ for the contralateral site $p > 0.05$).

Implications of this study for translational research

This study informs clinical trials by showing that 1-Hz rTMS delivered over area 22 in temporal cortex is safe and has a robust clinical effect in about half of subjects tested. VARL ratings of tinnitus loudness were more sensitive to the treatment effect of rTMS than were standardized measures of tinnitus severity like the TSI. PET imaging prior to treatment does not improve outcomes, in fact, it may be too variable within and between subjects to constitute a reliable targeting or outcome measure. Follow-up studies have shown that the effects of rTMS are reliable and suggest that repeating rTMS treatments as tinnitus returns—maintenance rTMS—may decrease tinnitus over time and delay its return [25]. Therefore, future treatment studies should also address a primary limitation of rTMS, which is its short-lived effect. Maintenance treatment represents an important future direction for rTMS investigations of tinnitus.

TMS INVESTIGATIONS OF DECISION-MAKING IN TOBACCO ADDICTION

Addiction is a chronic, compulsive disorder in which an individual continues to engage in a behavior (i.e., tobacco use, drug-taking, and gambling) despite negative consequences. The hallmark of an addictive disorder is relapse. Relapse involves choosing an immediately rewarding, impulsive option over an option that garners long-term rewards. This process is thought to be influenced by the endogenous reward-related processes in the brain [33]. rTMS applied to the prefrontal cortex affects reward-related decision-making [34,35]. Preliminary evidence suggests that high-frequency rTMS also affects cigarette smoking [36]. Our laboratory is currently testing the effects of rTMS on cigarette smoking and decision-making, particularly delay discounting, a type of reward-related decision-making known to be related to multiple addictive disorders, including cigarette smoking [33,37–40].

Given the hypothesized effects of rTMS on neuronal function, the effects of high-frequency rTMS delivered over prefrontal cortex on decision-making may be related to increased dopamine release in the endogenous reward system [41–43] as well as increases in arousal, sensory gating, and the ability to attend. (Animal studies show dopamine release following high-frequency rTMS, see Section "TMS investigations in rodents.") The following study is in the process of examining the effects of two levels of high-frequency stimulation to the dorsolateral prefrontal cortex (DLPFC) on decision-making in nonsmokers as well as 24-hour abstinent and nicotine-satiated smokers. The effects of rTMS on arousal, sensory gating, and attention are also examined. The internal validity of the study is enhanced by the inclusion of a valid control (sham) condition developed in our laboratory [3].

Methods

Participants (40 subjects: 20 smokers and 20 nontobacco users) aged 19–55 years who met eligibility criteria were enrolled. Smokers and nonsmokers receive three types of rTMS (10 Hz, 20 Hz, and sham) delivered over the left DLPFC guided by an MRI. Stimulations are separated by at least 48 hours. Subjects are assessed at baseline and immediately after stimulation. Smoking behaviors are tracked for 24 hours after stimulation.

Procedure

Baseline assessments are administered during a separate baseline assessment session. Smoking subjects in the acute withdrawal condition visit the laboratory 24 hours prior to the rTMS session, smoke one cigarette, and are instructed to refrain from administering any nicotine until after the rTMS session the next day. Salivary cotinine and exhaled CO levels are assessed. Upon returning to the lab 24 hours later, smoking subjects in the acute withdrawal condition are assessed for abstinence (exhaled CO, cotinine, and plasma nicotine). If they meet abstinence criteria, they receive stimulation. Upon arrival for stimulation, subjects in the satiated condition smoke one cigarette prior to receiving stimulation. All subjects receive active or sham rTMS delivered to the left DLPFC in a counterbalanced manner and guided by a magnetic resonance imaging (MRI) uploaded into the Brainsight system. Subjects receive a total of 900 pulses at each session at 110% of MT. In the 10-Hz active condition, they receive 90 ten-pulse trains (1-second on and 20-second off). In the 20-Hz condition, they receive 45 twenty-pulse trains (1-second on and 20-second off). The pulses in the sham condition mimic the 10-Hz condition.

Measures

A battery of widely used, objective measures are employed to assess (1) demographic characteristics, (2) smoking behaviors, history, dependence level, and withdrawal, (3) delay discounting, (4) arousal and sensory gating, and (5) attentional processes.

Decision-making

Measures of delay discounting were administered at baseline and after each of the three stimulation conditions (10 Hz, 20 Hz, and sham). The delay discounting tasks assess the degree to which rewards are modulated by the delay to their receipt [44]. Participants completed two tasks: $100 reward in hypothetical money and $1000 reward in hypothetical money. For each task, a series of choices were presented for each of seven delays: 1 day, 1 week, 1 month, 6 months, 1 year, 5 years, and 25 years. Smaller, immediately available rewards were offered against the larger constant delayed amount ($100 or $1000). The first choice was always between the larger delayed reward and half of the delayed reward available immediately. Subsequent choices adjust the immediate choice according to whether the participant chose the immediate or delayed reward. The final value at the end of the series is the indifference point for that delay. An indifference point is the value of the immediate reward, expressed as a proportion, subjectively deemed equivalent to the larger, delayed reward. The results for each task are expressed as the natural logarithm of k in Mazur's hyperbolic discounting model, with k increasing as the magnitude of the participant's preference for the smaller sooner reward increases [45]. The results from each task were also averaged to produce a mean delay discounting score. Data from existing published studies indicate values for log k range from about −12.00 to 4.00.

Arousal and sensory gating

The P50 auditory (click stimulus) evoked potential (AEP) is a measure of arousal recorded from the vertex of the head (Cz), generally occurring at a latency of 40–70 milliseconds in humans (see Chapter 3). Sensory gating can be quantified as the suppression ratio of the P50 AEP (decrease in from the first to second clicks in microvolts). The electrodes were placed at the vertex of the head (Cz) referenced to a frontal electrode (Fz). Eye movements (EOG, electroocculogram) were detected using diagonally placed canthal electrodes, while jaw movements (EMG, electromyogram) were detected using a lead over the masseter muscle referred to the chin. A subclavicular ground was used. Each channel is led to a Grass Instruments QP511 differential amplifier. The gain and bandpass were as follows: P50 potential × 50 K and 3 Hz to 1 kHz; EOG × 20 K and 3 Hz to 1 kHz; and EMG × 10 K and 30 Hz to 3 kHz, with a 60 Hz notch filter on each amplifier.

Participants were seated in a comfortable chair in a quiet room illuminated with bright light. Earphones were placed on participants and the hearing threshold for each ear determined using a Grass Instruments auditory stimulator STM10. Participants were instructed to keep their eyes open, gaze at the picture of a face placed on the wall four feet in front of them, and to count the number of paired clicks as a means of encouraging vigilance. The test stimulus was a rarefaction click of 0.1-millisecond duration set at least 50 dB above the hearing threshold delivered once every 5 seconds. Auditory stimulation consisted of paired clicks administered binaurally by headphones for 6–8 minutes or until 64 pairs of evoked potentials are acquired. The interstimulus interval was 250 milliseconds and the interpair interval was 5 seconds. The P50 AEP was administered at baseline and after the 10-Hz stimulation condition. While we focus on amplitude of the first P50 response, paired click stimuli allow us to explore latency of the first wave, time-to-peak, latency of the second wave, and habituation of the P50 amplitude to the second click. After amplification and filtering, signals were digitized at a sampling rate of 10 K samples per second using a National Instruments DAQCard 6036E, displayed, averaged and stored on a Dell Latitude using LABView software (National Instruments). All valid paired P50 evoked potentials for each participant were averaged. Electroencephalographic signals that contained interference from EOG or EMG were excluded from the average. Because the amplitude of the P50 potential is sleep state dependent, it is important to monitor vigilance with counts and by visual monitoring of the participant.

It should be noted that 64 trials yield an accurate and reproducible mean waveform for the majority of subjects. It requires a minimum of 6 minutes to acquire 64 trials for a P50 potential average.

Paired sample t-tests were used to test for significant differences between baseline and after stimulation on the latencies of the first and second waves, the time to peak (TTP) of the first and second waves, amplitude, and percent habituation. Independent sample t-tests were used to test for baseline differences between smokers and nonsmokers in these same variables.

Attentional processes

The psychomotor vigilance task (PVT) was utilized to measure attention and behavioral alertness. The PVT is a simple reaction time (RT) test that evaluates the ability to sustain attention and respond in a timely manner to salient signals [46]. Chapter 3 describes the method in detail. ANOVA was used to test for significant differences among conditions on the multiple performance parameters of the PVT.

Results

As hypothesized, our preliminary results indicate that high-frequency rTMS over the left DLPFC reduced delay discounting ($p = 0.02$). Post hoc tests revealed significant differences between baseline and 10 Hz ($p = 0.03$) and baseline and 20 Hz ($p < 0.005$); however, the difference between baseline and sham and between sham and 10 and 20 Hz was not significant (see Figure 4.3). Twenty-hertz stimulation had a greater effect on discounting than 10-Hz stimulation. It is presently unclear why sham did not differ from any of the other conditions. Significant differences were also found in measures of arousal. Stimulation (10 Hz) significantly decreased the mean latency to the first P50 potential ($t = 2.472$, df $= 39$, $p = 0.018$) and increased the TTP of the first P50 potential ($t = -2.359$, df $= 39$, $p = 0.023$), and the second P50 potential ($t = -3.054$, df $= 39$, $p = 0.004$). Our preliminary results also suggest that smokers and nonsmokers differ in the mean baseline amplitudes of the second wave (response to the second click) ($t = 0.443$, df $= 85$, $p = 0.005$). Stimulation appeared to have no effect on any of the performance parameters of the PVT. Analyses of the effects of stimulation on smoking behaviors, withdrawal, and craving are in process.

Implications for translational applications

If rTMS affects delay discounting in the expected direction, these results will contribute to the rationale that rTMS affects the activity of the DLPFC and perhaps the underlying endogenous reward system and may be incorporated as an effective component for the treatment of tobacco dependence as well as other addictive disorders.

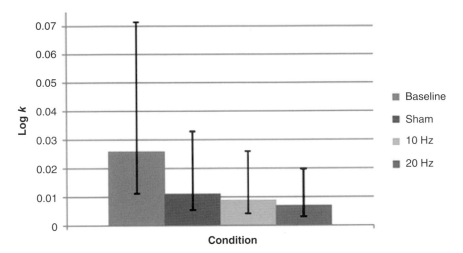

Figure 4.3   Delay discounting graphs. Discounting rate (k) by condition calculated using a hyperbolic-delay equation $v_d = V/(1 + kd)$, where v_d is the discounted value of a delayed reward, V is the objective value of the delayed reward, k is an empirically derived constant proportional to the degree of delay discounting, and d is delay duration. Main effect of condition $p = 0.02$; post hoc tests: baseline/10 Hz $p = 0.03$; baseline/20 Hz $p = 0.005$. (For color detail, please see the color plate section.)

TMS INVESTIGATIONS IN RODENTS

Optimization of rTMS in humans necessitates a broader knowledge of its evoked responses in brain tissue, which itself necessitates more fundamental study in animal models. However, rTMS research in rodents remains relatively sparse compared with human studies. For example, a Medline search of rTMS and human yielded 1164 articles, whereas a search of rTMS and rat yielded only 43 articles. However, reports indicate that rTMS is capable of altering rat brain function. For example, rTMS over the rat frontal cortex led to increased dopamine concentration in subcortical structures [43,47]. rTMS has also been reported to alter behavior in rodents. High-frequency rTMS (>1 Hz), administered daily in multiday paradigms, exhibited a pronounced antidepressant effect in the forced swim test model of depression [48–50]. However, reports of the anxiolytic properties of rTMS are inconsistent, with some reported improved performance in the plus-maze model of anxiety after prefrontal rTMS [51], while others report no rTMS-associated change in performance [48,52]. Low-frequency chronic rTMS has also been reported to inhibit spatial reference memory, as measured in the Morris water maze test [53].

There is evidence that rTMS on has a greater effect on some brain structures than on others. Ji et al. [54] reported that rTMS induced changes in c-fos mRNA expression in the dorsal midthalamus, hippocampus, pineal gland, and the frontal and cingulate cortices, but not in parietal cortex. Altering the position of the coil relative to the head did not alter this expression pattern [54]. Studies also suggest that rTMS is noncytotoxic in the rat; De Sauvage et al. used an alkaline comet assay to examine potential genotoxic effects of rTMS, and found no DNA damage following 10-Hz stimulation of frontal cortex [55].

By evaluating the effects of rTMS on specific behaviors (preattentional/arousal processing and sensory gating) in rats, our study provides an opportunity to gather significant new data about the physiological effects of rTMS and shed light on the mechanisms by which rTMS alters neural activity. To accomplish this, we are studying the effects of rTMS on an auditory evoked field potential, the rat P13 potential. In response to an auditory click stimulus, a positive waveform at a latency of 13 milliseconds can be recorded from the vertex of alert, freely moving rats. First described by Miyazato et al., a series of studies has established that the P13 potential is mediated by cholinergic neurons of the reticular activating system (RAS), specifically the pedunculopontine nucleus (PPN) [56–60]. The amplitude of the P13 potential is considered a measure of the level of arousal [56–60], and agents that decrease arousal also decrease P13 potential amplitude [59] (see also Chapter 6 for a complete description).

Sensory gating represents the critical function of filtering out extraneous information so that attention can be focused on newer, more salient stimuli. Sensory gating is often characterized by comparing the amplitudes of evoked responses elicited by repetitive stimuli. The ratio between the second (test) stimulus and the first (conditioning) stimulus is the "T/C ratio," has been used as a measure of sensory gating, and is used to measure habituation of responses to repeated stimuli. In humans, T/C ratios greater than ~0.5 are indicative of impaired gating, such as is in schizophrenia [61] anxiety disorder and depression [60]. In rats, we have shown that the T/C ratio of the P13 potential is impaired in pups born to dams exposed to cigarette smoke during pregnancy [62].

Even though TMS stimulates hundreds to thousands of neurons, studies of the motor cortex have shown that low-frequency stimulation (≤ 1 Hz) produces an inhibitory intermediate effect [14] whereas high-frequency stimulation (>5 Hz) produces intermediate excitatory effects [11,12]. The immediate goal of this research is to determine the optimal rTMS frequencies that lead either to a depression or an enhancement of the P13 auditory evoked potential and to evaluate the impact of rTMS on sensory gating. The knowledge gained from these experiments will be used to inform protocols focused on understanding the mechanisms by which rTMS may affect responses related to drug use and addiction, including dependency on nicotine and cigarettes.

Methods

Detailed description of surgical, recording, nicotine, and cigarette smoke administration protocols have been reported previously [59,63,64].

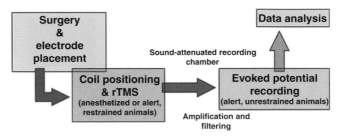

Figure 4.4 Protocol for TMS in animals. Diagram of the experimental protocol for TMS in animals. (For color detail, please see the color plate section.)

Figure 4.4 illustrates the experimental protocol. Briefly, animals are anesthetized and screw electrodes are placed over the vertex. After recovery, experimental manipulations (rTMS, drug administration, etc.) are performed and evoked potentials are recorded from alert unrestrained rats placed in a sound-attenuated and electrically shielded recording chamber.

rTMS therapy administration

In humans, TMS coils directly stimulate superficial cortex and the magnetic field can be focused on specific regions of the brain. However, in rats, deeper brain structures may be affected and the size of the rTMS coil relative to rat brain size prevents accurate focusing. The extent to which rTMS stimulation affects the rat brain is poorly characterized, but due to the relative disparity between the size of available coils and the rat brain it seems likely that using existing rTMS apparatus results in stimulation of a large proportion of the rat brain.

Results

rTMS administered to anesthetized animals

To establish the effects of rTMS exposure on the amplitude of the P13 potential, the appropriate rTMS protocol was determined empirically. Three variables were evaluated: (1) intensity of the magnetic field used during rTMS exposure, (2) frequency of rTMS, and (3) length of exposure. We determined that an intensity of 70% of maximum output, administered for 5 minutes at 1 Hz, produced a short-lived inhibition of P13 potential amplitude. For this experiment, animals were anesthetized with inhaled isoflurane during rTMS exposure and transferred to the recording chamber immediately after rTMS treatment. Potentials were recorded at 3 minutes intervals for 1 hour. Representative measurements of the amplitude of the conditioning response exposure to anesthesia and rTMS are shown in Figure 4.5. Comparison of this response to that elicited by anesthetic without rTMS shows that rTMS resulted in greater and longer lasting

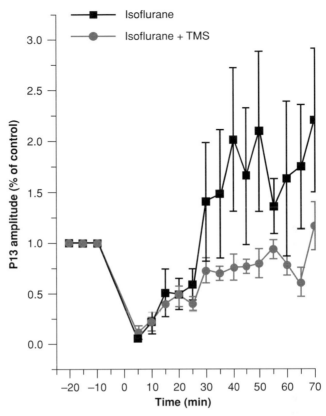

Figure 4.5 Effects of anesthesia and TMS on the P13 potential. Representative measurements of the amplitude of the conditioning response exposure to isoflurane anesthesia with and without rTMS. (For color detail, please see the color plate section.)

inhibition than anesthetic alone. rTMS treatment was followed by a short-lived (~10 minutes) return to pretreatment amplitude. In some cases, about 25 minutes after rTMS exposure ended, P13 potential amplitude was again inhibited for about 10 minutes. We cannot yet determine whether the increase in activity resulted from greater activity in the ascending output of the PPN (relayed by the thalamus to the cortex), or if this response was a result of direct activation of the thalamus or cortex. However, this observation suggests that, in rats at least, rTMS exposure has a significant effect on brain electrical activity and may be inducing oscillatory synchronization of cortical activity.

rTMS administered to alert animals

To prevent interference of the effects of anesthesia with the effects of rTMS, a procedure was developed for administering rTMS to alert animals.

For each TMS session, rats implanted with vertex electrodes were briefly anesthetized with isoflurane by inhalation. Anesthetized rats were placed in a soft, flexible restraint device and allowed to fully awaken for 15 minutes prior to stimulation. rTMS was administered for 20 minutes using a Magstim 87 mm figure-of-eight ventilated coil (Magstim Company Ltd, Carmarthenshire Wales, UK) at one of three randomly selected frequencies: (a) 1 Hz continuous stimulation, 1 click per second, 30% maximum machine output, 1200 pulses total, (b) 10-Hz three-pulse trains of 10 clicks per second and 3 seconds per train, with a 1-second delay between trains; delivered at 70% machine output (9000 pulses total), and (c) 20-Hz three-pulse trains of 20 clicks per second and 3 seconds per train, with a 1-second delay between trains; 70% machine output (18,000 pulses total). Each rat received rTMS once every 2 weeks. Rats received sham stimulation weekly, between rTMS sessions, using a Magstim 87 mm sham coil. During sham stimulation, animals were anesthetized, restrained, and allowed to recover for 15 minutes before sham stimulation began. The stimulating coil was placed nearby, but the rats were not subjected to the magnetic field produced; this was necessary to reproduce noise and restraint conditions present during rTMS administration.

In addition to single-day stimulations, rats were also given rTMS in five daily 20-Hz sessions (as described previously: 20 minutes per session three-pulse trains, 70% intensity), preceded and followed by a 2-day rest period and 3 days of pre- and poststimulation recordings. These experiments served to examine the effect of prolonged rTMS treatment and mirror an ongoing study of similar format in human subjects undergoing treatment for nicotine addiction.

Waveform measurements

Measurements of the amplitude of auditory evoked potentials were made from the beginning of the wave to its peak. If the baseline was not flat, then the beginning of the P13 potential was taken to be the change in slope of the recording occurring at 9–10-millisecond latency. Habituation of the P13 response was also calculated as a T/C ratio, with an increase in the T/C ratio indicating a decrease in habituation. This ratio is indicative of underlying neuronal system activity evoked by the stimulus and has been used as a measure of gating sensory stimuli. A recent study from our group showed a decrease in the habituation of the P13 potential in rats born to dams exposed to cigarette smoke during pregnancy [64]. To test habituation, a two stimulus paradigm was used in which the interstimulus interval is 0.5 second and the pairs of clicks were presented once every 5 seconds. The ratio of the amplitude of the P13 potential following the second (test) stimulus as a percentage of the amplitude of the P13 potential following the first (conditioning) stimulus served as a measure of habituation.

Statistics

Data were tested for normality using the Kolmogorov–Smirnov test for normality. Results were evaluated using two-factor repeated-measures ANOVA and main effects followed with post hoc contrasts using an appropriate posttest.

Results

Single rTMS in awake rats did not increase the P13 potential as expected (Figure 4.6). Since this could be attributed to interindividual variation and since rat studies suggest that multiple sessions of rTMS may induce changes in brain function where single sessions do not [64], we subjected the same rats to 5 days of daily stimulation at 20 Hz to mimic the conditions in an ongoing study examining rTMS on the P50 potential in cigarette smokers (Figure 4.7). Daily sessions, as measured in 3 days of posttesting following a 2-day rest period, also indicated no change in P13 potential relative to recordings from a 3-day pretest. We hypothesize that this may be due to the intrinsic properties of neurons of the RAS, which produce the P13 potential. If RAS neurons are already firing at their maximum rate in control rats, then excitatory stimulation will have no effect on P13 potential. However, it may act to restore or prevent decreases in sensory gating induced by nicotine.

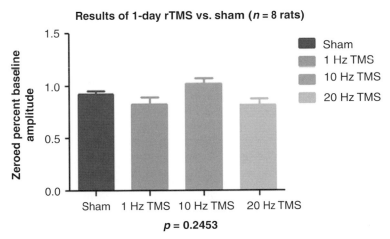

Figure 4.6   Effect of single-session rTMS on P13 potential amplitude. Note that TMS did not induce significant changes when applied at 1 Hz, 10 Hz, or 20 Hz, suggesting that TMS by itself does not alter the acute manifestation of the P13 potential. This establishes single-session TMS as a method that does not alter arousal, opening its use as a method to reduce or alter treatments that increase or decrease arousal levels. (For color detail, please see the color plate section.)

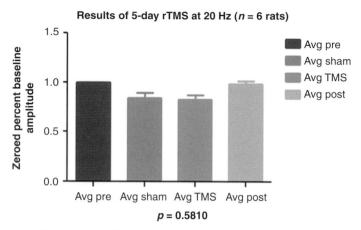

Results of 5-day rTMS at 20 Hz (*n* = 6 rats)

p = 0.5810

Figure 4.7   Effect of multiple session rTMS on P13 potential amplitude. Treatment with TMS similar to that used in humans (five daily rTMS sessions) failed to alter P13 potential amplitude in the rat compared with pre-TMS control or sham stimulation. In addition, P13 potential amplitude was not affected following rTMS, suggesting that multiple session TMS does not alter arousal, opening its use as a method to reduce or alter treatments that increase or decrease arousal levels. (For color detail, please see the color plate section.)

Future directions

Now that studies characterizing the effects of rTMS on the rat P13 potential have been completed, the effects of rTMS on responses to nicotine are being investigated. Nicotine has been shown to cause a temporary, but marked, dose-dependent decrease in the amplitude of the P13 potential [65]. Experiments to determine if rTMS alters this response are underway. Since rTMS appears to have no effect on the rat P13 potential in alert animals, it is likely that rTMS stimulation does not alter the results of the active neurons generating this potential. Since many of these neurons are already highly active, additional stimulation may not be capable of increasing their activity. However, because nicotine reduces neuronal activity, rTMS stimulation may restore the activities of these neurons, thereby modulating one of the primary effects of nicotine. Exploring the impact of rTMS stimulation on neurons whose activity has been inhibited will not only enhance understanding of the mechanisms by which rTMS exerts effects on neuronal activity, but will also provide a basis for developing models for applying rTMS to conditions in which neuronal activity is inhibited, including drug addiction. To better understand the potential long-term effects of rTMS treatments, we are also investigating the effects of rTMS on gene expression of ion channels, neurotransmitter receptors, and inflammatory markers using real-time quantitative polymerase chain reaction (RT-qPCR) arrays.

CONCLUSION

By using the rat as an rTMS model the ability to investigate mechanisms underlying its effects at the behavioral, cellular and molecular levels. This model has the potential to bridge the gap between cellular and human studies, thus representing a truly integrative, translational approach to developing rTMS as a useful therapeutic intervention.

REFERENCES

1. Smith J, Mennemeier M, Bartel T, Chelette KC, Kimbrell TA, Triggs W, Dornhoffer JL. (2007) Repetitive transcranial magnetic stimulation for tinnitus: a pilot study. Laryngoscope 117, 529–534.
2. Richter GT, Mennemeier M, Bartel T, Chelette KC, Kimbrell TA, Triggs W, Dornhoffer JL. (2006) Repetitive transcranial magnetic stimulation for tinnitus: a case study. Laryngoscope 116, 1867–1872.
3. Mennemeier M, Triggs W, Chelette KC, Woods AJ, Kimbrell TA, Dornhoffer JL. (2009) Sham transcranial magnetic stimulation using electrical stimulation of the scalp. Brain Stimul: Basic, Translate Clin Res Neuromodulin 2, 168–173.
4. Wagner T, Valero-Cabre A, Pascual-Leone A. (2007) Noninvasive human brain stimulation. Annu Rev Biomed Eng 9, 527–565.
5. Bohning DE. (2000) Introduction and overview of TMS physics. In: George MS, Belmaker RH, eds. Transcranial Magnetic Stimulation in Neuropsychiatry. Washington, DC: American Psychiatric Press, pp. 13–44.
6. Roth BJ MS. (1994) Algorithm for the design of magnetic stimulation coils. Med Biol Eng Comput 32, 214–216.
7. Cohen LG, Roth BJ, Nilsson J, Dang N, Panizza M, Bandinelli S, Friauf W, Hallett M. (1990) Effects of coil design on delivery of focal magnetic stimulation. Technical considerations. Electroenceph Clin Neurophysiol 75, 350–357.
8. George MS, Nahas Z, Kozel FA, Li X, Denslow S, Yamanaka K, Mishory A, Foust MJ, Bohning DE. (2002) Mechanisms and state of the art of transcranial magnetic stimulation. J ECT 18, 170–181.
9. Bear, MF. (1999) Homosynaptic long-term depression: a mechanism for memory? Proc Natl Acad Sci USA 96, 9457–9458.
10. Stanton, PK. (1989) Associative long-term depression in the hippocampus induced by hebbian covariance. Nature 339, 215–218.
11. Pascual-Leone A, Meador KJ. (1998) Is transcranial magnetic stimulation coming of age? J Clin Neurophysiol 15, 285–287.
12. Wu T, Sommer M, Tergau F, Paulus W. (2000) Lasting influence of repetitive transcranial magnetic stimulation on intracortical excitability in human subjects. Neurosci Lett 287, 37–40.
13. Malenka RC, Nicoll RA. (1999) Long-term potentiation: a decade of progress? Science 285, 1870–1874.

14. Chen R, Classen J, Gerloff C, Celnik P, Wassermann EM, Hallett M, Cohen LG. (1997) Depression of motor cortex excitability by low-frequency transcranial magnetic stimulation. Neurology 48, 1398–1403.

15. Fitzgerald, PB, Brown TL, Marston NA, Daskalakis ZJ, De Castella A, Kulkarni J. (2003) Transcranial magnetic stimulation in the treatment of depression: a double-blind, placebo-controlled trial. Arch Gen Psychiatry 60, 1002–1008.

16. Avery DH, Holtzheimer PE 3rd, Fawaz W, Russo J, Neumaier J, Dunner DL, Haynor DR, Claypoole KH, Wajdik C, Roy-Byrne P. (2006) A controlled study of repetitive transcranial magnetic stimulation in medication-resistant major depression. Biol Psychiatry 59, 187–194.

17. O'Reardon J, Solvason H, Janicak P, Sampson S, Isenberg K, Nahas Z, McDonald W, Avery D, Fitzgerald P, Loo C, Demitrack M, George M, Sackeim H. (2007) Efficacy and safety of transcranial magnetic stimulation in the acute treatment of major depression: a multisite randomized controlled trial. Biol Psychiatry 62, 1208–1216.

18. Klein E, Kreinin I, Chistyakov A, Koren D, Mecz L, Marmur S, Ben-Shachar D, Feinsod M. (1999) Therapeutic efficiency of right prefrontal slow repetitive transcranial magnetic stimulation in major depression: a double blind controlled trial. Arch Gen Psychiatry 56, 315–320.

19. Rossi S, Ferro M, Cincotta M, Ulivelli M, Bartalini S, Miniussi C, Giovannelli F, Passero S. (2007) A real electro-magnetic placebo (REMP) device for sham transcranial magnetic stimulation (TMS). Clinical Neurophysiology 118, 709–716.

20. Coles RR. (1987) Epidemiology of Tinnitus. Edinburgh: Churchill Livingstone, pp. 46–70.

21. Kadner A, Viirre E, Wester DC, Walsh SF, Hestenes J, Vankov A, Pineda JA. (2002) Lateral inhibition in the auditory cortex: an EEG index of tinnitus? NeuroReport 13, 443–446.

22. Jastreboff PJ, Gray WC, Gold SL. (1996) Neurophysiological approach to tinnitus patients. Amer J Otol 17, 236–240.

23. Muhlnickel W, Elbert T, Taub E, Flor H. (1998) Reorganization of auditory cortex in tinnitus. Proc Natl Acad Sci USA 95, 10340–10343.

24. Rauschecker J. (1999) Auditory cortical plasticity: a comparison with other sensory systems. Trends Neurosci 22, 74–80.

25. Mennemeier M, Chelette KC, Myhill J, Taylor-Cooke P, Bartel T, Triggs W, Kimbrell T, Dornhoffer J. (2008) Maintenance repetitive transcranial magnetic stimulation can inhibit the return of tinnitus. Laryngoscope 118, 1228–1232.

26. Llinas R. (2001) The I of the Vortex, from Neurons to Self. Cambridge: MIT Press.

27. Rossi S, De Capua A, Ulivelli M, Bartalini S, Falzarano V, Filippone G, Passero S. (2007) Effects of repetitive transcranial magnetic stimulation on chronic tinnitus: a randomised, crossover, double blind, placebo controlled study. J Neurol Neurosurg Psychiatry 78, 857–863.

28. Plewnia C, Reimold M, Najib A, Reischl G, Plontke SK, Gerloff C. (2007) Moderate therapeutic efficacy of PET-navigated transcranial magnetic stimulation against chronic tinnitus: a randomised, controlled pilot study. J Neurol Neurosurg Psychiatry 78, 152–156.

29. Kleinjung T, Eichhammer P, Langguth B, Jacob P, Marienhagen J, Hajak G, Wolf SR, Strutz J. (2005) Long-term effects of repetitive transcranial magnetic stimulation (rTMS) in patients with chronic tinnitus. Otolaryngol Head Neck Surg 132, 566–569.

30. Langguth B, De Ridder D, Dornhoffer JL, Eichhammer P, Folmer RL, Frank E, Fregni F, Gerloff C, Khedr E, Kleinjung T, Landgrebe M, Lee S, Lefaucheur JP, Londero A, Marcondes R, Moller AR, Pascual-Leone A, Plewnia C, Rossi S, Sanchez T, Sand P, Schlee W, Pysch D, Steffens T, van de Heyning P, Hajak G. (2008) Controversy: does repetitive transcranial magnetic stimulation/transcranial direct current stimulation show efficacy in treating tinnitus patients? Brain Stimulation 1, 192–205.

31. Mennemeier M, Chelette KC, Allen S, Bartel TB, Triggs W, Kimbrell T, Crew J, Munn T, Brown GJ, Dornhoffer J. (2011) Variable changes in PET activity before and after rTMS treatment for tinnitus. Laryngoscope 121, 815–822.

32. Landgrebe M, Binder H, Koller M, Eberl Y, Kleinjung T, Eichhammer P, Graf E, Hajak G, Langguth B. (2008) Design of a placebo-controlled, randomized study of the efficacy of repetitive transcranial magnetic stimulation for the treatment of chronic tinnitus. BMC Psychiatry 8, 23.

33. Bickel WK, Miller ML, Yi R, Kowal BP, Lindquist DM, Pitcock JA. (2007) Behavioral and neuroeconomics of drug addiction: competing neural systems and temporal discounting processes. Drug Alcohol Depend 90(suppl 1), S85–S91.

34. Knoch D, Fehr E. (2007) Resisting the power of temptations: the right prefrontal cortex and self-control. Ann N Y Acad Sci 1104, 123–134

35. Knoch D, Gianotti LR, Pascual-Leone A, Treyer V, Regard M, Hohmann M, Brugger P. (2006) Disruption of right prefrontal cortex by low-frequency repetitive transcranial magnetic stimulation induces risk-taking behavior. J Neurosci 26, 6469–6472.

36. Eichhammer P, Johann M, Kharraz A, Binder H, Pittrow D, Wodarz N, Hajak G. (2003) High-frequency repetitive transcranial magnetic stimulation decreases cigarette smoking. J Clin Psychiatry 64, 951–953.

37. Bickel WK, Marsch LA. (2001) Toward a behavioral economic understanding of drug dependence: delay discounting processes. Addiction 96, 73–86.

38. Bickel WK, Odum AL, Madden GJ. (1999) Impulsivity and cigarette smoking: delay discounting in current, never, and ex-smokers. Psychopharmacology 146, 447–454.

39. Bickel WK, Yi R, Kowal BP, Gatchalian KM. (2008) Cigarette smokers discount past and future rewards symmetrically and more than controls: is discounting a measure of impulsivity? Drug Alcohol Depend 96, 256–262.

40. Baker F, Johnson MW, Bickel WK. (2003) Delay discounting in current and never-before cigarette smokers: similarities and differences across commodity, sign, and magnitude. J Abnorm Psychol 112, 382–392.

41. Murase S, Grenhoff J, Chouvet G, Gonon FG, Svensson TH. (1993) Prefrontal cortex regulates burst firing and transmitter release in rat mesolimbic dopamine neurons studied in vivo. Neurosci Lett 157, 53–56.

42. Karreman M, Moghaddam B. (1996) The prefrontal cortex regulates the basal release of dopamine in the limbic striatum: an effect mediated by ventral tegmental area. J Neurochem 66, 589–598.

43. Erhardt A, Sillaber I, Welt T, Muller MB, Singewald N, Keck ME. (2004) Repetitive transcranial magnetic stimulation increases the release of dopamine in the nucleus accumbens shell of morphine-sensitized rats during abstinence. Neuropsychopharmacology 29, 2074–2080

44. Logue AW. (1988) Research on self-control: An integrating framework. Behav Brain Sci 11, 665–709.

45. Mazur JE. (1987) An adjusting procedure for studying delayed reinforcement. In: Commons ML, Mazur JE, Nevin JA, Rachlin H, eds. Quantitative Analysis of Behavior. Hillsdale, NJ: Erlbaum, pp. 55–73.

46. Dorrian J, Rogers NL, Dinges DF. (2005) Psychomotor vigilance performance: a neurocognitive assay sensitive to sleep loss. In: Kushida CA, ed. Sleep Deprivation: Clinical Issues, Pharmacology and Sleep Loss Effects. New York, NY: Marcel Dekker Inc., pp. 39–70.

47. Keck, ME, Welt T, Müller MB, Erhardt A, Ohl F, Toschi N, Holsboer F, Sillaber I. (2002) Repetitive transcranial magnetic stimulation increases the release of dopamine in the mesolimbic and mesostriatal system. Neuropsychopharmacology 43, 101–109.

48. Keck ME, Engelmann M, Müller MB, Hennigan MSH, Hermann B, Rupprecht R, Neumann ID, Toschi N, Landgraf R, Post A. (2000) Repetitive transcranial magnetic stimulation induces active coping strategies and attenuates the neuroendocrine stress response in rats. J Psychiatric Res 34, 265–276.

49. Tsutsumi T, Fujiki M, Akiyoshi J, Horinouchi Y, Isogawa K, Hori S, Nagayama H. (2002) Effect of repetitive transcranial magnetic stimulation on forced swimming test. Prog Neuropsychopharmacol Biol Psychiatry 26, 107–111.

50. Kim EJ, Kim WR, Chi SE, Lee KH, Park EH, Chae J-H, Park SK, Kim HT, Choi J-S. (2006) Repetitive transcranial magnetic stimulation protects hippocampal plasticity in an animal model of depression. Neurosci Lett 405, 79–83.

51. Kanno M, Matsumoto M, Togashi H, Yoshioka M, Mano Y. (2003) Effects of acute repetitive transcranial magnetic stimulation on extracellular serotonin concentration in the rat prefrontal cortex. J Pharmacol Sci 93, 451–457.

52. Hargreaves GA, McGregor IS, Sachdev PS. (2005) Chronic repetitive transcranial magnetic stimulation is antidepressant but not anxiolytic in rat models of anxiety and depression. Psychiatry Res 137, 113–121.

53. Li W, Yang Y, Ye Q, Yang B, Wang Z. (2007) Effect of chronic and acute low-frequency repetitive transcranial magnetic stimulation on spatial memory in rats. Brain Res Bull 71, 493–500.

54. Ji R-R, Schlaepfer TE, Aizenman CD, Epstein CM, Qiu D, Huang JC, Rupp F. (1998) Repetitive transcranial magnetic stimulation activates specific regions in rat brain. Proc Natl Acad Sci USA 95, 15635–15640.

55. De Sauvage RC, Lagroye I, Billaudel B, Veyret B. (2008) Evaluation of the potential genotoxic effects of rTMS on the rat brain and current density mapping. Clin Neurophysiol 119, 482–491.

56. Miyazato H, Skinner RD, Reese NB, Boop FA, Garcia-Rill E. (1995) A middle latency auditory evoked potential in the rat. Brain Res Bull 37, 247–255.

57. Miyazato H, Skinner RD, Garcia-Rill E. (1999) Sensory gating of the P13 midlatency auditory evoked potential and the startle response in the rat. Brain Res 822, 60–71.

58. Miyazato H, Skinner RD, Garcia-Rill E. (1999) Neurochemical modulation of the P13 midlatency auditory evoked potential in the rat. Neuroscience 92, 911–920.

59. Miyazato H, Skinner RD, Cobb M, Andersen B, Garcia-Rill E. (1999) Midlatency auditory evoked potentials in the rat—effects of interventions which modulate arousal. Brain Res Bull 48, 545–553.

60. Garcia-Rill E, Skinner RD, Clothier J, Dornhoffer J, Uc E, Fann A, Mamiya N. (2002) The sleep state-dependent midlatency auditory evoked P50 potential in various disorders. Thalamus Relat Syst 2, 9–19.

61. Freedman R, Adler LE, Gerhardt GA, Waldo M, Baker N, Rose GM, Drebing C, Nagamoto H, Bickford-Wimer P, Franks R. (1987) Neurobiological studies of sensory gating in schizophrenia. Schizophrenia Bull 13, 669–678.

62. Garcia-Rill E, Buchanan R, McKeon K, Skinner RD, Wallace T. (2007) Smoking during pregnancy: postnatal effects on arousal and attentional brain systems. NeuroToxicology 28, 915–923.

63. Mamiya N, Buchanan RA, Skinner RD, Garcia-Rill, E. (2005) Nicotine suppresses the P13 auditory evoked potential by acting on the pedunculopontine nucleus in the rat. Exp Brain Res 164, 109–119.

64. Garcia-Rill E, Wallace-Huitt T, Mennemeier M, Charlesworth A, Heister D, Ye M, Yates, C. (2008) Neuropharmacology of pediatric and adult sleep and wakefulness. In: Lee-Chiong TL, ed. The Wiley Guide to Sleep Medicine: A Concise Reference and Review. Hoboken, NJ: Wiley.

5 Translational Studies in Drug Abuse

Veronica Bisagno, William E. Fantegrossi, and Francisco J. Urbano

BACKGROUND AND SIGNIFICANCE

The ultimate purpose of the research supported through our translational funding initiative is to support a broad array of translational studies linking basic neuroscience and treatments for drug abusing populations (with and without comorbid psychiatric disorders) across the spectrum of abused drugs. Findings from research on the neurobiological, neurocognitive, and neurobehavioral processes that are associated with substance abuse may provide drug abuse treatment researchers with important data and new approaches for developing and/or adapting treatment interventions for substance use disorders. Similarly, a clearer understanding of the specific neurobiological effects and the mechanism of action of abused substances may lead to the modification of existing therapies or may lead to the development of more efficacious treatments for drug-addicted individuals that translate into sustainable changes in behavior.

Prominent features of drug addiction can be modeled in laboratory animals with increasing validity and reliability, thereby allowing detailed investigations of the relevant mechanisms involved. From a clinical perspective, drug addiction continues to exact enormous human and economic costs on society, yet available treatments are inadequate for most people. An improved understanding of the molecular and cellular mechanisms underlying drug addiction will lead to better treatments. In this regard, from a basic neuroscience perspective, studies of the neurobiology of drug addiction offer a unique opportunity to establish the biological basis of a complex and clinically relevant behavioral abnormality.

Psychostimulant addiction is one of the most intractable disorders encountered by health care professionals, but translational research into the mechanisms by which cocaine (for example) exerts its reinforcing and

Translational Neuroscience: A Guide to a Successful Program, First Edition. Edited by Edgar Garcia-Rill.
© 2012 John Wiley & Sons, Inc. Published 2012 by John Wiley & Sons, Inc.

rewarding effects has been fruitful. Cocaine acts on the mesoaccumbens dopamine (DA) pathway of the midbrain, extending from the ventral tegmental area to the nucleus accumbens [1,2]. This pathway is also known as the "reward pathway" as it is the area of the brain that is activated when someone has a pleasurable experience such as eating, sex, or receiving praise [1,3]. (However, it is important to note that objectively aversive experiences such as electric shock [4], tail pinch [5], physical restraint [6], and social defeat [7] can also increase DA neurotransmission in this region, suggesting that the often-applied "reward pathway" appellation is almost certainly too simplistic and, perhaps, misleading.)

In DA neurotransmission, a transmitting neuron releases DA that then binds to DA receptors on the receiving neuron; ultimately leading to the propagation of an action potential in the receiving neuron. After this has occurred, cell surface DA reuptake transporters (DATs) of the transmitting cell pump the DA back into the cell to be repackaged in vesicles and used again. Cocaine binds to these DATs, thus blocking them from functioning. As a result, DA levels increase in the synapse, and consequently, the receiving neuron is continuously stimulated. This constant firing of the neurons leads to a feeling of euphoria. In addicts, cocaine blocks between 60% and 77% of the DAT binding sites; in order to attain a "high," at least 47% of the binding sites must be blocked by cocaine [8]. Cocaine also acts on the reuptake transporters of serotonin and norepinephrine, and therefore, the levels of these neurotransmitters are also increased [9]. Increased synaptic serotonin may modulate the euphoric effects of psychostimulants, as reuptake inhibitors with pronounced serotonergic effects are less reinforcing and rewarding in animals models as compared to more DA selective compounds [10]. Similarly, serotonin selective reuptake inhibitors lack reinforcing and rewarding effects in animal models, and in humans using these drugs as antidepressants. Norepinephrine stimulates the "fight or flight" response of the sympathetic nervous system characterized by heightened heart rate, blood pressure, respiration rate, and body temperature as well as dilation of pupils and sweating; these phenomena produce an energizing feeling. Although serotonin and norepinephrine certainly contribute to the interoceptive effects of cocaine, numerous lines of research all converge on the conclusion that it is the effects of cocaine on central DA that determine its abuse potential [11].

At a certain point, cocaine usage ceases to be a voluntary action: this is the onset of addiction. It is thought that repeated exposure to cocaine alters neurochemistry and neurotransmission such that strong feelings of drug craving are induced, and these cravings seem to drive more and more behaviors toward obtaining and using the drug [12]. Animal models have been used to investigate the effects of cocaine on reinforcement and associative learning, and, more recently, animal models of drug craving have been exploited to probe the neurobiology of addiction.

Since cocaine craving is often triggered by environmental stimuli previously associated with drug use [13], the role of drug-paired cues in cocaine addiction has become an active area of research. An interesting and useful animal model in this regard is known as place conditioning, or conditioned place preference (CPP), wherein the distinct contextual cues of a testing chamber (floor texture, patterns on chamber walls, shape of chamber, etc.) are associated with cocaine or placebo administration. When rodents are allowed to freely roam between these environments after experiencing repeated conditioning sessions confined to the cocaine- and placebo-paired contexts, they will come to spend more time in the environment where they were administered the drug. This demonstrates that the contextual cues paired with cocaine have acquired appetitive stimulus properties (which elicit approach behavior) through their association with drug administration. Animals thus express a "preference" for an environment consisting of these cues to by increasing the amount of time they spend in that cocaine-paired environment, as compared to a similar context-rich environment that presumably remains motivationally neutral through its association with placebo. A decrease in time spent in the drug-paired context is termed a "conditioned place aversion" and may indicate that the conditioning drug has aversive stimulus properties [14]. CPP continues to be one of the most popular models to study the motivational effects of drugs [15], and the conditioned effects of drugs are thought to contribute to their abuse liability [16]. Furthermore, the CPP assay is not technically challenging, and automated chambers or video-tracking behavior recognition software allow for objective measures to be obtained.

Many regions of the brain express DA receptors and DA transporters, and are thus susceptible to cocaine effects. In recent years, there has been significant progress made in imaging methods including positron emission tomography (PET) and functional magnetic resonance imaging (fMRI) that have led to the discovery of differences between regional activations in addicts and healthy control subjects [17]. Particular interest has focused on frontal and parietal or somatosensory cortex, amygdala, several portions of the striatum and the thalamus. Thalamus and cortex together with neostriatal areas are massively interconnected [18,19]. In rodents, the somatosensory thalamus is populated by two distinct sets of elements: (1) cortically projecting relay cells such as ventrobasal (VB) neurons that subserve the thalamocortical loop via glutamatergic synapses on middle layers of the somatosensory cortex and (2) reticular thalamic GABAergic neurons projecting to and inhibiting VB neurons. Cortical layer V and VI pyramidal neurons subserve the corticothalamic loop via glutamatergic synapses directly on both reticular and VB thalamic nuclei [19].

Chronic consumption of stimulants is associated with major clinical complications [20]. In particular, excessive cocaine use may cause seizures [21] and cerebral hypoxia [20]. Cocaine-induced delirium can sometimes be associated with such perceptual distortions as hallucinations, suggesting cocaine-mediated abnormal thalamocortical processing [22]. In a visuospatial attention task, using fMRI, cocaine abusers showed lower thalamic activation, higher occipital and prefrontal cortex activation, and higher deactivation of parietal regions compared with controls [17]. Thus, use of neuroimaging and other techniques during adolescence may characterize specific neurobiological incentive-motivational circuitry that may be involved in emotional regulation, drug seeking, addiction, reward, relapse, and maintenance of behavioral change, and may identify new targets for therapeutic interventions. In this regard, we have shown that in vivo electroencephalographic recordings in adolescent mice receiving a cocaine dose regimen designed to model a "binge" (three injections at 15 mg/kg/injection, administered at 1-hour intervals) showed a significant increment in low frequencies without concomitant changes in high-frequency gamma-band activity. In vitro patch recordings from VB neurons after cocaine "binge" administration showed low threshold spike activation at more negative membrane potentials and increases in both h-currents and low voltage activated T-type calcium currents. Also, a 10-mV negative shift of the threshold activation level of T-type currents and a significant increase in both frequency and amplitude of GABA-A receptor-mediated miniature membrane potentials were observed. In conclusion, our data indicate that thalamocortical dysfunctions observed in cocaine abusers might be due to two distinct but additive events: (1) increased low frequency oscillatory thalamocortical activity and (2) overinhibition of VB neurons that can abnormally "lock" the whole thalamocortical system at low frequencies [23]. Further characterization of other psychostimulant effects on thalamocortical networks is still lacking.

BEHAVIORAL CORE FACILITY

We routinely perform systems-level studies using state-of-the art behavioral equipment that is available to most research centers and universities. These automated systems allow us to share information, protocols, and even replicate results from other laboratory settings where this technology is also available. This fact will increase the opportunities for networking, discussing new insights, and improving training in cutting edge behavioral techniques for doctoral and postdoctoral students. Importantly, our capacity for behavioral testing is multimodal, including place conditioning, drug discrimination, drug self-administration, and assays of drug-elicited behaviors. This breadth of analysis allows us to ask multidimensional questions, use behavioral tests that are specifically suited to answer these questions, and, most importantly, to establish translational research programs that approach our topics from the molecular to the behavioral level.

Behavioral tests in psychostimulant abuse

Automated video tracking: Ethovision

Conditioned place preference

CPP (or, more simply, place conditioning) is a commonly used test to assess preferences for environmental stimuli that have been associated with drug administration. CPP involves repeated conditioning sessions where the animal is presented with the drug while confined to a distinct environment containing various cues, and trials where the animal is administered the drug vehicle and confined to a different contextual environment. Later on, when animals are tested in the drug-free state, entries into and overall amount of time spent in the compartment previously associated with the drug can be quantified as measures of reward learning, where the learned association between environmental stimuli and drug effect presumably provides the basis for CPP experiments.

We use a three-compartment CPP apparatus that provides visual (black dots vs. gray stripes), tactile (rough floor vs. grid floor), and geometric cues (square compartment with four corners vs. multiangled polygon compartment) for the two conditioning compartments, which are connected by a smooth transparent polycarbonate hallway. General activity and location in the apparatus is monitored by video recording from above, and total time in each compartment is recorded using Ethovision XT 7.0 (Noldus Inc., USA).

Experimental procedure for CPP

Phase 1: Habituation phase

On two 30-minute sessions (1 session/day), mice are able to freely explore the entire apparatus. This phase is designed to minimize novelty-induced locomotor stimulation, which might otherwise interfere with assessment of initial preference.

Phase 2: Preconditioning bias test

To determine whether a preexisting *bias* for one chamber or the other exists in each experimental subject, a single 30-minute test session is conducted during which mice are allowed to freely explore both conditioning chambers. The time spent in each of the conditioning arenas is recorded (as is time in the neutral "hallway"), and time spent in each chamber is evaluated to determine initial preference and aid group assignments. We typically counterbalance our groups such that equal numbers of subjects receive drug in each compartment and always assign drug conditioning to the *nonpreferred* arena.

Phase 3: Conditioning

A total of four 30-minute conditioning sessions are used for each mouse. Subjects receive drug in the assigned chamber, and saline in the other chamber, on alternate days. No behaviors are recorded during these conditioning trials. Mice are simply injected, placed into their conditioning chamber, and allowed to associate the interoceptive effects of the injection with the environmental cues of the conditioning arena.

Phase 4: Postconditioning bias test

A single 30-minute preference tests is conducted 24 hours after the last conditioning session. The conditions of these tests are identical to those during the preconditioning bias test, in that mice are placed into the apparatus in a drug-free state and allowed to freely explore both conditioning chambers. The amount of time spent in the previously drug-paired compartment is measured and the results are compared with those from the preconditioning bias test.

Sensorimotor tests: combining locomotor activity with single cell patch-clamp recordings from the same animals

Addictive psychostimulants derive a major part of their reinforcing impact by activating brain mechanisms associated with normal behaviors such as exploratory behavior and locomotor activity. Locomotor activation often corresponds with psychostimulant reinforcement [9,24]. Importantly, locomotor activity is easy to measure, making this a frequently used test for preliminary determination of experimental manipulations that may affect psychostimulant addiction. Locomotor activity has been also used to study the conditioning and the adaptive responses that occur after repeated psychostimulant administration, which often produce locomotor sensitization (i.e., an increase in the locomotor response to the same dose of drug as a consequence of repeated administration).

Despite the relative ease with which locomotor activity can be collected and quantified, it should be noted that there are important variables to consider when designing an experiment using motor activity as an endpoint. For example, a subject's familiarity with the testing environment can have profound effects on motor behavior, with novel environments eliciting greater degrees of motor stimulation than more familiar environments [25]. Housing conditions of the subjects can also impact both basal locomotor activity and locomotor responses to psychostimulant drugs. For example, rats living in isolated conditions displayed enhanced locomotor activity on exposure to a novel environment, in comparison to rats housed in an enriched environment, and this difference was further exaggerated following administration of either amphetamine or cocaine [26]. Suffice it to say that the relative ease of *collecting* locomotor data should not blind researchers to the fact that the experimental *design* of such experiments must be approached carefully.

In our facilities, locomotor tests are typically performed in an open field to which the animal was previously exposed in order to allow exploration and habituation. Software like Ethovision XT (Noldus Inc., USA) allows the consecutive recording of up to six boxes (e.g., "arenas"), in which both saline- and psychostimulant-injected subjects can be analyzed simultaneously. Data collected from these sessions include time length in which the animals walk, jump, sniff, and so on.

One example of this test used in a drug abuse research protocol is a study aimed at exploring the role of T-type calcium channels on cocaine-induced hyperlocomotion. In this study, we were able to demonstrate that T-type calcium channels play a key role in cocaine-mediated behavioral responses and GABAergic thalamocortical alterations [27]. Patch clamp recordings of GABAergic mini-inhibitory postsynaptic currents (IPSCs) of VB neurons in slices were obtained from mice after the administration of 2-octanol (i.p., 0.5 mg/kg, 30 minutes before first and third cocaine injections)+saline, mibefradil (i.p., 20 mg/kg, 90 minutes before first injection)+saline, 2-octanol (i.p., 0.5 mg/kg, 30 minutes before first and third injections)+cocaine "binge," and mibefradil (i.p., 20 mg/kg, 90 minutes before first injection)+cocaine "binge." When compared to saline alone, both 2-octanol and mibefradil preadministration did not affect basal GABAergic mini-IPSC frequency (Figure 5.1A). However, a drastic reduction in frequency was observed when both T-type calcium channel blockers were combined with a cocaine "binge" regimen of drug administration (Figure 5.1B). On average, GABAergic mini-IPSC interevent intervals were significantly longer (i.e., lower frequencies) for the combination of 2-octanol+cocaine "binge" (Figure 5.1C, solid blue circles), and mibefradil+cocaine "binge" (Figure 5.1C, solid green circles) compared to cocaine "binge" alone (Figure 5.1C, filled red circles [27]).

We then studied in vivo the effects of mibefradil (i.p., 20 mg/kg) and 2-octanol (i.p., 0.07 mg/kg) on locomotor stimulation induced by the cocaine "binge." The average distance traveled by mice increased after each individual cocaine injection in the "binge" protocol (Figure 5.1D and E, solid red circles), while it remained unaffected by saline injections alone (Figure 5.1D and E, solid gray circles). Mibefradil coadministration reduced the cocaine-induced hyperlocomotion at 20 mg/kg (Figure 5.1D). Likewise, 2-octanol coadministration reduced cocaine-induced hyperlocomotion (Figure 5.1E). These results strongly suggest that T-type calcium channels can be considered key elements for cocaine-mediated locomotor effects. Furthermore, in vitro patch-clamp recordings obtained from mice previously administered locomotor stimulant doses of cocaine represent a novel approach for translational studies in drug abuse.

Automated gait analysis: CatWalk

There are several assisted automated gait analysis systems that provide a comprehensive method to assess a number of dynamic and static gait parameters simultaneously. These automated systems are available to investigate significant deficits in locomotor performance. One of these systems

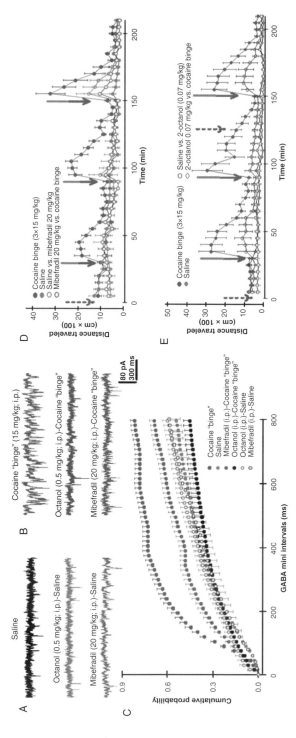

Figure 5.1 Cocaine-induced involvement of *T*-type calcium channels in thalamocortical GABAergic transmission. Coadministration of *T*-type calcium channel blockers prevented cocaine-mediated enhancement of GABAergic transmission onto VB neurons in vivo. Representative GABAergic mini currents in VB neurons recorded from mice injected with saline ((A) without and with previous in vivo i.p. injections of 2-octanol 0.5 mg/kg or mibefradil 20 mg/kg) or cocaine ((B) 3 × 15 mg/kg, 1 hour apart and with 2-octanol 0.5 mg/kg and mibefradil 20 mg/kg). (C) Average cumulative probability plots of GABAergic mini interevent intervals recorded in VB neurons from mice injected with all combinations showed in (A) and (B). Note how GABAergic mini interevent intervals were significantly affected by in vivo administration of *T*-type calcium blockers 2-octanol and mibefradil (see the text). (D) Mibefradil reduced cocaine-induced hyperlocomotion. Plot showing the average distance traveled (in cm × 100) by mice i.p.-injected with saline (gray-filled circles), cocaine (red-filled circles), saline pretreated with mibefradil (empty gray circles) and cocaine pretreated with mibefradil (empty green circles). (E) Same as (D), for 2-octanol (0.07 mg/kg). (For color detail, please see the color plate section.)

is CatWalk (Noldus Inc., Leesburg, VA), which uses video images of the animals' paws acquired with a high-speed video camera to detect individual footprints and to quantify the animals' weight distribution using a fluorescent light this system within a narrow corridor. This system is often used in protocols of spinal cord injury, cerebellar ataxia, and stroke. However, recent findings indicate that the motor consequences of even brief exposures to psychostimulant drugs can persist long after the stimulant is discontinued. We are currently evaluating locomotor disturbances in psychostimulant exposed rodents using the CatWalk system, and believe this technique to be quite useful in the study of functional consequences of long-term psychostimulant intake in animal models.

Voltage-sensitive dye imaging

Voltage-sensitive dye imaging (VSDI) is an optical fluorescence imaging technique that offers the possibility to visualize, in real time, the cortical activity of large neuronal populations with high spatial resolution (down to 20–50 μm) and high temporal resolution (down to the millisecond). With such resolution, VSDI appears to be the best technique to study the dynamics of cortical processing at the neuronal population level. Experiments using VSDI to assess how profound and how long-lasting cocaine effects are on GABAergic networks are underway.

There is a VSDI assembly for slices from juvenile mice (Figure 5.2). This equipment allows us to combine patch-clamp and extracellular population recordings simultaneously with acquisition of VSDI images using an Evolve 512 EMCCD camera (Figure 5.2, right upper photo) (see Chapter 3). Thalamocortical interactions can be analyzed in slices stained with the voltage-sensitive dye di-4 ANEPPS [28]. Fluorescence from the whole somatosensory cortex can be simultaneously acquired with population responses during low (10 Hz) and high (40 Hz) frequency stimulation of afferents from VB thalamus [19]. Future VSDI experiments will help us assess how profound and how long-lasting cocaine (and other psychostimulant) effects are on thalamocortical glutamatergic and GABAergic networks. Also, the possible protective role of modafinil will also be investigated, expanding current knowledge on a potentially effective pharmacological tool to prevent and/or arrest the deleterious effects of cocaine as well as other psychostimulants on thalamocortical networks and the behaviors they modulate.

Intravenous drug self-administration

Behaviorism proposes that the actions of an organism are governed by their consequences according to principles of operant conditioning [29], and the term reinforcement is used to describe the relationship between

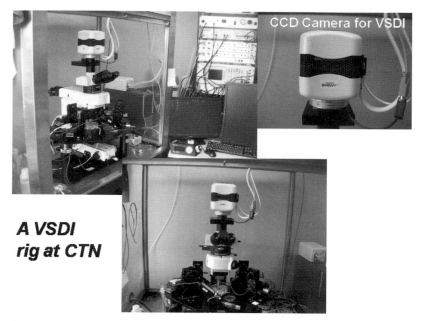

Figure 5.2 Photomicrographs showing voltage-sensitive dye imaging (VSDI) and patch clamp rig. Upper left image shows low-magnification photograph of the voltage sensitive dye rig. Upper right image shows detailed photograph of the Evolve camera used for VSDI recordings. Middle lower photograph shows micromanipulator arrangement and interface chamber used for VSDI experiments located on top of a Gibraltar stage in combination with an upright microscope. (For color detail, please see the color plate section.)

a behavior and its consequences. Drug self-administration is a technique that allows for the study of drug reinforcement, as the operant response directly produces administration of the pharmacological substance. Such experiments assess the reinforcing effects of a drug by quantifying an increase in the frequency of the behavior that produces drug administration. One critical factor in establishing and maintaining behavior under a given set of contingencies is immediacy of reinforcer delivery, and when studying drugs as reinforcers, this can sometimes pose problems. Essentially, experimenters ask laboratory animals to associate their behavior (for example, the depression of a response lever) with some change in interoceptive state induced by drug administration. Ideally, this change in interoceptive state should occur as rapidly after drug administration as possible in order to facilitate such an association. To the extent that different routes of drug administration can influence onset of drug action, a majority of researchers using drug self-administration procedures have chosen to use intravenous preparations in order to maximize the speed with which drug effects are induced, although it should be noted that delivery of some compounds via intramuscular [30], inhalation [31], and oral [32] routes also maintain behavior. In laboratory animals, intravenous preparations involve the surgical insertion of an indwelling venous catheter (typically into a jugular vein) that is then routed subcutaneously to the midscapular region. From here, the catheter either exits the animal and passes through a "tether" system [33,34], or connects to a subcutaneously implanted vascular access port [35,36]. In either case, the catheter can then be attached to a drug supply via an electronic infusion pump, the operation of which is controlled by the behavior of the animal according to experimenter-determined schedule contingencies.

Drug self-administration studies in animals have contributed substantially to our knowledge of the neuropharmacological mechanisms controlling drug abuse. For example, studies with opioids have shown that drugs with high affinity for μ-opioid receptors function as positive reinforcers [37,38], whereas opioids with high affinity for κ-opioid receptors generally do not [37,39]. Additionally, the self-administration of psychomotor stimulants and opioids has been found to be affected by the administration of antagonists either systemically or centrally [40,41]. If administration of an antagonist shifts the dose–response function for a self-administered drug to the right, then it can be assumed that the site of action of the antagonist is important for the reinforcing effects of the drug [42,43]. In addition to the administration of antagonists, self-administration of drugs has been affected by lesions of certain brain neurotransmitter systems [40,41]. Studies have also found that animals will self-administer drugs directly into certain brain areas, suggesting a neuropharmacological mechanism for their reinforcing effects [40].

Over the years, drug self-administration procedures in animals have been found to be valid and reliable for determining the abuse liability of drugs in humans, as it is well established that animals will self-administer most drugs that are abused by humans [44,45]. The primary focus of drug self-administration research in laboratory animals has been to establish the reinforcing properties of drugs of abuse and to identify neurochemical mechanisms underlying drug use. A better understanding of the neurochemical basis of drug self-administration is essential for the development of treatment medications for human drug abusers. Toward that end, a number of control procedures have been described to demonstrate that increases in behavior that result in drug delivery are caused specifically by the reinforcing effects of the drug [46]. The most commonly used procedure is to substitute saline for the drug solution and determine whether the behavior undergoes extinction. The rate and pattern of responding maintained by drug delivery depends on a number of variables including the schedule of reinforcement, drug dose, the volume and duration of injection, and the duration of drug self-administration sessions. Drug self-administration studies have consistently obtained an inverted U-shaped dose-effect curve relating the unit dose of drug delivered per injection and response rate or number of injections delivered. The dose-effect function likely reflects a combination of reinforcing effects and unconditioned stimulus effects such as sedation or marked hyperactivity. Typically, the ascending limb of the dose-effect curve reflects the reinforcing effects, and response rate increases with drug dose. In contrast, the descending limb of the curve probably reflects a nonspecific disruption of operant behavior as excessive drug accumulates over the session, and response rate decreases with drug dose. It should be noted that the dose-effect curve relating the unit dose of drug delivered per injection and drug intake in mg/kg is typically a monotonic increasing function. Lastly, an inverse relationship has been obtained between infusion duration and reinforcing effects [47,48], such that the longer the infusion time required to deliver a constant volume of drug solution, the less effectively the drug functions as a reinforcer. However, this relationship is typically not observed until the infusion duration is extended to a minute or more.

Animal models of drug self-administration provide a rigorous, systematic approach to characterize the reinforcing effects of psychoactive drugs. Research efforts that have used these models of drug self-administration have focused primarily on the identification of neurochemical mechanisms that underlie drug reinforcement, and the development of pharmacotherapies to treat drug addiction. In clinical evaluations of new medications, a decrease in drug self-administration is the goal of treatment [49–51]. Preclinical evaluations of pharmacotherapies require the establishment of stable baseline patterns of drug self-administration prior to drug-interaction studies. Subsequently, the treatment medication is administered as a pretreatment before the conduct of self-administration sessions. It is critical to study several doses of the treatment medication to determine an effective dose range and a maximally effective dose that lacks overt behavioral toxicity. The effects of the treatment medication typically are evaluated first in combination with a dose of the self-administered drug on the ascending limb of the dose-effect curve that maintains high rates of self-administration. However, a complete dose-effect curve should be characterized for the self-administered drug because pretreatment effects can differ depending on the unit dose of the drug self-administered. A rightward shift in the dose-effect curve suggests that drug pretreatment is antagonizing the reinforcing effects of the self-administered drug. A downward displacement of the dose-effect curve indicates an insurmountable attenuation of the reinforcing effects. Alternatively, a leftward shift is consistent with an enhancement of the reinforcing effects. Medications that shift the dose-effect curve downward and decrease self-administration over a broad range of unit doses are most likely to have therapeutic utility. Medications that shift the dose-effect curve to the right and simply alter the potency of the self-administered drug may prove to be ineffective at higher unit doses of self-administered drug. Clinically, most medications are administered on a chronic basis and may require long-term exposure before therapeutic effects are noted [52]. Accordingly, preclinical studies should include repeated daily exposure to the medication to characterize peak effectiveness and to document continued effectiveness over multiple sessions [53]. It is also critical to reestablish baseline levels of drug self-administration between successive exposures to the medication to ensure that the catheter preparation is functional and that persistent effects of the pretreatment drug do not interfere with the interpretation of drug interactions obtained.

The primary treatment outcome measures in drug self-administration studies are rate of responding and the number of drug injections delivered per session. Both measures are influenced by the schedule of reinforcement, drug dose, the volume and duration of injection, and the duration of the self-administration session. Moreover, most drugs that are self-administered have direct effects on rate of responding that may be distinct from their reinforcing effects. For example, cocaine injections may increase rate of responding early in the session, but suppress behavior later in the session as total drug intake accumulates. Another important consideration in evaluating medication effectiveness is the selectivity of effects on drug self-administration. If the drug pretreatment decreases drug self-administration at lower doses or to a greater extent than behavior maintained by a nondrug reinforcer such as food, the outcome is indicative of selective interactions with the reinforcing properties of the self-administered drug. In contrast, a nonspecific disruptive effect on operant behavior will likely suppress drug- and food-maintained responding to a comparable extent. Lastly, the reinforcing properties and abuse potential of the medication should be evaluated by substituting a range of doses of the medication for the self-administered drug. Since reinforcing effects in preclinical studies are correlated with abuse liability in humans, reliable self-administration of the medication is usually considered undesirable.

REFERENCES

1. Wise RA. (1985) The anhedonia hypothesis: Mark III. Behav Brain Sci 8, 178–186.
2. Torres GE, Gainetdinov RR, Caron MG. (2003) Plasma membrane monoamine transporters: structure, regulation and function. Nat Rev Neurosci 4, 13–25.
3. Kelley AE, Berridge KC. (2002) The neuroscience of natural rewards: relevance to addictive drugs. J Neurosci 22, 3306–3311.
4. Abercrombie E, Keefe K, DiFrischia D, Zigmond M. (1989) Differential effect of stress on in vivo dopamine release in striatum, nucleus accumbens and medial frontal cortex. J Neurochem 52, 1655–1658.
5. Louilot A, Le Moal M, Simon H. (1986) Differential reactivity of dopaminergic neurons in the nucleus accumbens in response to different behavioral situations. An in vivo voltammetric study in free moving rats. Brain Res 397, 395–400.
6. Imperato A, Angelucci L, Casolini P, Zocchi A, Puglisi-Allegra S. (1992) Repeated stressful experiences differently affect limbic dopamine release during and following stress. Brain Res 577, 194–199.

7. Tidey JW, Miczek KA. (1996) Social defeat stress selectively alters mesocorticolimbic dopamine release: an in vivo microdialysis study. Brain Res 721, 140–149.

8. Volkow ND, Wang GJ, Fischman MW, Foltin RW, Fowler JS, Abumrad NN, Vitkun S, Logan J, Gatley SJ, Pappas N, Hitzemann R, Shea CE. (1997) Relationship between subjective effects of cocaine and dopamine transporter occupancy. Nature 386, 827–830.

9. Wise RA, Bozarth MA. (1987) A psychomotor stimulant theory of addiction. Psychol Rev 94, 469–492.

10. Czoty PW, Ginsburg BC, Howell LL. (2002) Serotonergic attenuation of the reinforcing and neurochemical effects of cocaine in squirrel monkeys. J Pharmacol Exp Ther 300, 831–837.

11. Howell LL, Kimmel HL. (2008) Monoamine transporters and psychostimulant addiction. Biochem Pharmacol 75, 196–217.

12. Weiss F, Ciccocioppo R, Parsons LH, Katner S, Liu X, Zorrilla EP, Valdez GR, Ben-Shahar O, Angeletti S, Richter RR. (2001) Compulsive drug-seeking behavior and relapse. Neuroadaptation, stress, and conditioning factors. Ann N Y Acad Sci 937, 1–26.

13. Childress AR, Hole AV, Ehrman RN, Robbins SJ, McLellan AT, O'Brien CP. (1993) Cue reactivity and cue reactivity interventions in drug dependence. NIDA Res Monogr 137, 73–95.

14. Bardo MT, Bevins RA. (2000) Conditioned place preference: what does it add to our preclinical understanding of drug reward? Psychopharmacology 153, 31–43.

15. Tzschentke TM. (2007) Measuring reward with the conditioned place preference (CPP) paradigm: update of the last decade. Addict Biol 12, 227–462.

16. Tzschentke TM. (1998) Measuring reward with the conditioned place preference paradigm: a comprehensive review of drug effects, recent progress and new issues. Prog Neurobiol 56, 613–672.

17. Tomasi D, Goldstein RZ, Telang F, Maloney T, Alia-Klein N, Caparelli EC, Volkow ND. (2007) Thalamo-cortical dysfunction in cocaine abusers: implication in attention and perception. Psychiatry Res: Neuroim 155, 189–201.

18. Wright AK, Norrie L, Ingham CA, Hutton EA, Arbuthnott GW. (1999) Double anterograde tracing of outputs from adjacent "barrel columns" of rat somatosensory cortex. Neostriatal projection patterns and terminal ultrastructure. Neuroscience 88, 119–133.

19. Llinás RR, Leznik E, Urbano FJ. (2002) Temporal binding via cortical coincidence detection of specific and nonspecific thalamocortical inputs: a voltage-dependent dye-imaging study in mouse brain slices. Proc Natl Acad Sci USA 99, 449–454.

20. Devlin RJ, Henry JA. (2008) Clinical review: major consequences of illicit drug consumption. Crit Care 12, 202.

21. Hanson GR, Jensen M, Johnson M, White HS. (1999) Distinct features of seizures induced by cocaine and amphetamine analogs. Eur J Pharmacol 377, 167–173.

22. Behrendt RP. (2006) Dysregulation of thalamic sensory "transmission" in schizophrenia: neurochemical vulnerability to hallucinations. J Psychopharmacol 20, 356–372.

23. Urbano FJ, Bisagno V, Wikinski SI, Uchitel OD, Llinas RR. (2009). Cocaine acute "binge" administration results in altered thalamocortical interactions in mice. Biol Psychiatry 66, 769–776.
24. Kuczenski R, Segal DS. (1992) Differential effects of amphetamine and dopamine uptake blockers (cocaine, nomifensine) on caudate and accumbens dialysate dopamine and 3-methoxytyramine. J Pharmacol Exp Ther 262, 1085–1094.
25. Badiani A, Anagnostaras SG, Robinson TE. (1995) The development of sensitization to the psychomotor stimulant effects of amphetamine is enhanced in a novel environment. Psychopharmacology (Berl) 117, 443–452.
26. Smith JK, Neill JC, Costall B. (1997) Post-weaning housing conditions influence the behavioural effects of cocaine and d-amphetamine. Psychopharmacology (Berl) 131, 23–33.
27. Bisagno V, Raineri M, Peskin V, Wikinski SI, Uchitel OD, Llinás RR, Urbano FJ. (2010) Effects of T-type calcium channel blockers on cocaine-induced hyperlocomotion and thalamocortical GABAergic abnormalities in mice. Psychopharmacology (Berl) 212, 205–214.
28. Llinás R, Urbano FJ, Leznik E, Ramírez RR, van Marle HJ. (2005) Rhythmic and dysrhythmic thalamocortical dynamics: GABA systems and the edge effect. Trends Neurosci 28, 325–333.
29. Skinner BF. (1938). The Behavior of Organisms. New York: Appleton-Century-Crofts.
30. Goldberg SR, Morse WH, Goldberg DM. (1976) Behavior maintained under a second-order schedule by intramuscular injection of morphine or cocaine in rhesus monkeys. J Pharmacol Exp Ther 199, 278–286.
31. Carroll ME, Krattiger KL, Gieske D, Sadoff DA. (1990) Cocaine-base smoking in rhesus monkeys: reinforcing and physiological effects. Psychopharmacology (Berl) 102, 443–450.
32. Gomez TH, Roache JD, Meisch RA (2002) Orally delivered alprazolam, diazepam, and triazolam as reinforcers in rhesus monkeys. Psychopharmacology (Berl) 161, 86–94.
33. Yanagita T, Deneau GA, Seevers MH. (1963) Methods for studying psychogenic dependence to opiates in the monkey. Committee on Drug Addiction and Narcotics, NRCNAS, Ann Arbor, MI.
34. Schuster CR, Thompson T. (1963) A technique for studying self-administration of opiates in Rhesus monkeys. Committee on Drug Addiction and Narcotics, NRCNAS, Ann Arbor, MI.
35. Carroll ME. (1994) Pharmacological and behavioral treatment of cocaine addiction: animal models. NIDA Res Monogr 145, 113–130.
36. Wojnicki FH, Bacher JD, Glowa JR. (1994) Use of subcutaneous vascular access ports in rhesus monkeys. Lab Anim Sci 44, 491–494.
37. Young AM, Stephens KR, Hein DW, Woods JH. (1984) Reinforcing and discriminative stimulus properties of mixed agonist-antagonist opioids. J Pharmacol Exp Ther 229, 118.
38. France CP, Winger GD, Medzihradsky F, Seggel MR, Rice KC, Woods JH. (1991) Mirfentanil: Pharmacological profile of a novel fentanyl derivative with opioid and nonopioid effects. J Pharmcol Exp Ther 258, 502.

39. Tang AH, Collins RJ. (1985) Behavioral effects of a novel kappa-opioid analgesic, U-50488, in rats and rhesus monkeys. Psychopharmacology (Berl) 85, 309.

40. Koob GF, Bloom FE. (1988) Cellular mechanisms of drug dependence. Science 242, 715.

41. Koob GF, Weiss F. (1990) Pharmacology of drug self-administration. Alcohol 7, 193.

42. Wilson MC, Schuster CR. (1972) The effects of chlorpromazine on psychomotor stimulant self-administration in the rhesus monkey. Psychopharmacology (Berl) 26, 115.

43. Dewit H, Wise RA. (1977) Blockade of cocaine reinforcement in rats with the dopamine receptor blocker pimozide, but not with the noradrenergic blockers phentol-amine or phenoxybenzamine. Can J Psychol 31, 195.

44. Mello NK. (1979) Behavioral pharmacology of narcotic antagonists. In: Peterson RC, ed. The International Challenge of Drug Abuse, NIDA Research Monograph Series 19. Washington, DC: US Government Printing Office, pp. 126–141.

45. Griffiths RR, Bigelow GE, Henningfield JE. (1980) Similarities in animal and human drug-taking behavior. In: Mello NK, ed. Advances in Substance Abuse 1. Greenwich, CT: JAI Press, pp. 1–90.

46. Pickens R, Thompson T. (1968) Cocaine-reinforced behavior in rats: effects of reinforcement magnitude and fixed-ratio size. J Pharmacol Exp Ther 161, 122.

47. Balster RL, Schuster CR. (1973) Fixed-interval schedule of cocaine-reinforcement: effect of dose and infusion duration. J Exp Anal Behav 20, 119.

48. Kato S, Wakasa Y, Yanagita T. (1987) Relationship between minimum reinforcing doses and injection speed in cocaine and pentobarbital self-administration in crab-eating monkeys. Pharmacol Biochem Behav 28, 407.

49. Mello NK, Mendelson JH. (1980) Buprenorphine suppresses heroin use by heroin addicts. Science 27, 657.

50. Mello NK, Mendelson JH, Bree MP. (1981) Naltrexone effects on morphine and food self-administration in morphine-dependent rhesus monkeys. J Pharmacol Exp Ther 218, 550.

51. Mello NK, Mendelson JH, Kuehnle JC. (1982) Buprenorphine effects on human heroin self-administration. J Pharmacol Exp Ther 230, 30.

52. Gawin FH, Ellinwood EH. (1988) Cocaine and other stimulants: Actions, abuse and treatment. N Engl J Med 318, 1173.

53. Negus SS, Mello NK. (2003) Effects of chronic d-amphetamine treatment on cocaine- and food-maintained responding under a second-order schedule in rhesus monkeys. Drug Alcohol Depend 70, 39.

6 Electrophysiology in Translational Neuroscience

Edgar Garcia-Rill

In this chapter, we deal with complementary electrophysiological methods that can (a) investigate the same process in animal models, and (b) extend the human electrophysiology approaches beyond the electroencephalography (EEG) and evoked potential studies described in Chapter 3.

IN VIVO AND IN VITRO ANIMAL MODELS

In Chapter 3, we described the design of an Electrophysiology Core Facility and detailed studies using the midlatency auditory evoked P50 potential as a measure of level of arousal and of habituation to repetitive input. This quantitative assessment of brainstem-thalamus processing allows one to quickly and noninvasively secure information about processes that, if disturbed, will impact higher processing such as attention and selective attention, and, if undisturbed, will allow one to determine if attentional and selective attentional processes are independently disrupted. However, one can design an Animal Electrophysiology Core Facility to be able to perform parallel and concurrent studies of arousal and habituation in vivo and in vitro. That is, one can perform studies on freely moving animals and in animal brain slices, and target the same brain centers involved in generating the P50 potential in humans. The rodent equivalent of the P50 potential in man is the P13 potential, which has the same characteristics of sleep state-dependence, rapid habituation, and modulation by cholinergic agents. We can study the amplitude of the P13 potential as a measure of level of arousal in the freely moving rat, and use a paired stimulus paradigm to investigate habituation to repetitive stimulation or sensory gating in awake animals [1]. Since we know that the P50 potential and the P13 potential are modulated by the pedunculopontine nucleus (PPN), one

Translational Neuroscience: A Guide to a Successful Program, First Edition. Edited by Edgar Garcia-Rill.
© 2012 John Wiley & Sons, Inc. Published 2012 by John Wiley & Sons, Inc.

can develop a research program using brainstem slices containing the PPN to inform us about the cellular and molecular organization of this region. Combined with the study of PPN cellular and molecular mechanisms in vitro, we can, therefore, address changes in the P13 potential at the level of the whole animal, and correlate these to the human equivalent, the P50 potential. This allows one to study processes detected in vitro, confirmed in the whole animal, and tested in humans.

MODAFINIL

One example of a process we can study in vitro, in vivo, and in homo is the action of the atypical stimulant modafinil. In the rat, the waveforms following an auditory stimulus are the brainstem auditory evoked response (BAER), the P7 potential at 7-millisecond latency, the P13 potential at 13-millisecond latency, and the P25 potential at 25-millisecond latency. The midlatency auditory evoked P13 potential appears to be the rodent equivalent of the human P50 potential and the feline "wave A" [2]. It is the only midlatency auditory evoked response that has the same three characteristics as the human P50 potential and feline "wave A" as described above. Since the P13 potential can be elicited after decerebration, or after ablation of the primary auditory cortex bilaterally, it appears to have a subcortical origin. Convincing evidence for the subcortical origin of the vertex-recorded P13 potential is that injections of various neuroactive agents known to inhibit PPN neurons, when injected into the posterior midbrain in the rat, will reduce or block the P13 potential, while not affecting the primary auditory P7 potential. Noradrenergic, GABAergic, serotonergic, and cholinergic agents are all know to inhibit PPN neurons, and injection of each of these agents in the region of the PPN reduced or blocked the P13 potential in a dose-dependent manner. Moreover, interventions that modulate arousal such as various anesthetics, head injury and ethanol, all selectively reduced or blocked the P13 potential in a dose-dependent manner (reviewed in reference [2]).

PPN neurons, many of which are cholinergic, increase firing during waking ("Wake-on") and rapid eye movement (REM) sleep ("REM-on"), or both ("Wake/REM-on"), but decrease firing significantly during slow-wave sleep, suggestive of increased excitation during activated states, exactly like the P50 potential in humans and the P13 potential in rodents. The following describes how findings in single cells in the PPN in vitro led to the testing of a novel stimulant on the P13 potential in whole animals, with parallel effects on the P50 potential in humans. These studies allow the design of studies transitioning easily between the bench, the bedside, and back to the bench. Novel mechanisms for the control of sleep and waking promise to lead to the development of new stimulants and anesthetics.

PATCH CLAMP RECORDINGS

Patch clamp recordings is a technique that involves placing tissue slices in a submersion chamber that is fed temperature-controlled oxygenated cerebrospinal fluid. The chamber lies on the stage of a microscope such as the Nikon FN-1 upright fluorescence microscope, and the tissue can be visualized with water-immersion lenses such that single cells can be observed (at 400 × amplification). A patch microelectrode is brought into contact with the selected cell and a seal formed using suction such that the electrode forms a high-resistance seal on the surface, then the membrane is ruptured so that the intracellular fluid is continuous with the microelectrode solution. The cell can then be "clamped" using current or voltage. This technique allows one to test intrinsic membrane properties as well as to test membrane responses to pharmacological agents, from the firing of action potentials, to changes in the membrane potential, to the opening and closing of single channels on the membrane (cell attached mode without rupturing the membrane). This technology has been extensively used in neuroscience research, and a number of studies relevant to the processes we have been considered can be drafted.

For example, the presence of electrical coupling in the PPN was discovered several years ago [3]. Dye coupling was detected between cells (injection of dye into one cell passively diffused to another through gap junctions), and these studies determined that pairs of PPN cells were electrically coupled (current steps applied to one cell were evident in the other cell in the presence of the sodium channel blocker tetrodotoxin—TTX, that eliminates action potentials, and coupling was blocked by gap junction blockers). This work also detected protein levels and mRNA of the neuronal gap junction protein connexin 36 (Cx-36). Punches (1-mm diameter punches from brainstem slices) of the nucleus in question were analyzed for Cx-36 protein. This study showed that Cx 36 was present at high levels early in development (10 days of age) and decreased dramatically during the developmental decrease in REM sleep (30 days). The decrease was evident in all of the reticular activating system (RAS) nuclei analyzed (PPN, sub-coeruleus (SubC), and intralaminar thalamus/parafascicular (Pf) nucleus).

Modafinil is approved for the treatment of excessive daytime sleepiness in narcolepsy, daytime sleepiness due to obstructive sleep apnea, and to shift work sleep disorder, and is also prescribed in a number of neuropsychiatric conditions. The literature on this agent acknowledges that the mechanism of action of modafinil is unknown, although it has been found to increase glutamatergic, adrenergic, and histaminergic transmission and to decrease GABAergic transmission. Modafinil was found to increase electrical coupling between cortical, thalamic reticular, and inferior olive neurons [4]. Following pharmacologic blockade of connexin permeability, modafinil restored electrotonic coupling. The effects of modafinil were counteracted by the gap junction blocker mefloquine. It has been proposed that modafinil may increase electrotonic coupling and in which case the high input resistance typical of GABAergic neurons is reduced. Modafinil was also found to increase electrical coupling in the RAS by decreasing the input resistance of electrically coupled RAS cells, an effect blocked by the gap junction antagonists carbenoxolone or mefloquine [3]. These studies proposed that increased electrical coupling of GABAergic RAS neurons by modafinil may decrease their input resistance and, consequently, GABA release, thus disinhibiting output cells, perhaps accounting for its stimulant properties. The fact that its mechanism of action is through disinhibition, makes it a better option than other stimulants like amphetamine, that activate addiction pathways and thus have significant abuse potential. The presence of electrical coupling in the RAS, which may act with known transmitter interactions to generate ensemble activity, provides new and exciting directions for the field of sleep-wake control.

Studies were then designed to determine if injections of modafinil into the PPN would affect the amplitude of the P13 potential in the awake, freely moving rat, and if its stimulant effects were blocked by gap junction antagonists [5]. Modafinil injected into the PPN increased arousal levels in a dose-dependent manner as determined by the amplitude of the P13 potential in the rat, an effect blocked by the gap junction antagonists mefloquine and carbenoxolone, suggesting that one mechanism by which modafinil increased arousal may have been by increasing electrical coupling. The fact that the anesthetics halothane and propofol are known to block gap junctions and also to induce anesthesia, make this finding relevant for the field of anesthesia.

Studies on the human P50 potential showed that oral modafinil increased the amplitude of the P50 potential, confirming that the amplitude of this waveform can be used as a measure of arousal level in the human. The same effect, that is, increased amplitude, was observed in the vertex-recorded auditory midlatency P13 potential after oral administration in the rat, while a similar increase in amplitude of the P13 potential was observed after intracranial administration of modafinil into the region of the PPN [1]. The use of parallel preparations, the human P50 potential, the rodent P13 potential, and brainstem slices, allow investigation of arousal systems in humans as well as invasive/interventional studies in animals on the same neurological substrate. Animal models of a number of disorders can be used to study changes in P13 potential characteristics that parallel those of the human P50 potential in the same disorder.

GAMMA BAND ACTIVITY

During waking and paradoxical sleep, the EEG is characterized by low amplitude, high frequency activity in the gamma band range ($\sim$30–90 Hz). Gamma frequency oscillations appear to participate in sensory perception, and such coherent events may occur at cortical or thalamocortical levels. Similar oscillations have been described in the hippocampus and cerebellum. The question arises, is there gamma band activity in the RAS? Do PPN neurons exhibit gamma band activity in terms of action potential frequency of single cells, and/or does the population as a whole show gamma band activity when pharmacologically activated, and/or does the cholinergic input increase the frequency of these oscillations? Amazingly, recent patch clamp experiments found that the maximal firing frequency in all PPN neurons was in the gamma range. Moreover, PPN neurons showed gamma oscillations when voltage-clamped at holding potentials above −25 mV, indicating their origin is spatially located beyond voltage clamp control. The cholinergic agonist carbachol (CAR) was found to increase the frequency of the oscillations. The N-type calcium channel blocker w-conotoxin-GVIA partially reduced gamma oscillations, while the P/Q-type blocker w-agatoxin-IVA abolished them. The delayed rectifier-like potassium channel blocker α-dendrotoxin also abolished gamma oscillations. These results identified the mechanism underlying the generation of gamma band oscillations in the PPN. It was also the first time that the potential roles of high voltage-activated calcium, and voltage-gated potassium channels had been described in oscillations in PPN cells. There is now little doubt that PPN neurons also have the ability to manifest gamma band activity that is enhanced by cholinergic input, such as that reported in cortical, thalamic, hippocampal, and cerebellar cells. Moreover, PPN neurons appear to oscillate at gamma band through P/Q-, and N-type calcium channels, as well as voltage-gated, delayed rectifier-like, potassium channels, suggesting that multiple mechanisms may modulate these cells to fire at gamma band frequencies [6].

In addition, it was found that a descending target of the PPN, the SubC nucleus that is involved in REM sleep signs, and an ascending target, the intralaminar Pf nucleus that is involved in cortical activation, also manifest gamma band activity, the former through sodium-dependent subthreshold oscillations, and the latter through P/Q-type calcium channels. These studies showed that elements of the RAS all manifest gamma band activity (Figure 6.1). Gamma band activity in the cortex is thought to persist for hundreds of milliseconds or even seconds. How does a circuit maintain such rapid, recurrent activation? Expecting a circuit of, say, five or ten synapses to reliably relay 30–80 Hz cycling without failing is unrealistic. Central synapses, even those in primary sensory pathways, hardly follow more than 20-Hz stimulation. Without the intrinsic properties afforded by rapidly oscillating channels, gamma band activity could not be maintained for long. Thus, the combination of channels capable of fast oscillations and circuitry that involves activating these channels is a more likely scenario for the maintenance of gamma band oscillations. As far as the PPN is concerned, as part of the RAS, one would expect it to be activated by all sensory modalities, and to relay such activation to ascending targets

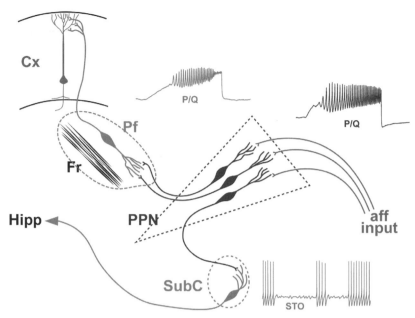

Figure 6.1 **Gamma band activity in the reticular activating system (RAS).** Wiring diagram of RAS nuclei manifesting gamma band activity and the mechanisms behind these oscillations. Afferent input that originates from collateral activation of the RAS by sensory systems activates the dendrites of pedunculopontine nucleus (PPN) neurons. The presence of P/Q- and N-type calcium channels in the dendrites set off oscillations at gamma band that influence firing frequency. The output of the PPN descends to the subcoeruleus (SubC), presumably activating these neurons that have sodium-dependent subthreshold oscillations. These cells in turn influence downstream systems involved in the atonia of REM sleep, and ascending systems that may participate in the consolidation of memories such as the hippocampus (Hipp). The output of the PPN also ascends to the intralaminar thalamus, especially the parafascicular (Pf) nucleus, activating its dendrites to oscillate at gamma frequency via P/Q- and N-type calcium channels. These cells in turn project to the cortex, particularly to upper cortical layers where the nonspecific thalamic inputs terminate, to activate cortical neurons. Once cortical, hippocampal, and cerebellar cells are activated, the generation and maintenance of gamma band activity in the brain can more easily be maintained. (For color details, please see the color plate section.)

such as the Pf nucleus to induce cortical synchronization of fast activity, and descending targets such as the SubC nucleus involved in paradoxical sleep signs. Figure 6.1 is a diagram of the RAS nuclei exhibiting gamma band activity.

POPULATION RESPONSES

Another way of recording activity that is intermediate between evoked responses such as the P13 potential and single cell activity such as that determined using whole cell patch clamp recordings is the use of population responses. You need to use an interface chamber (instead of a submersion chamber like in patch clamp) to record population responses in the PPN after application of transmitters known to modulate the PPN. The reason is that the overlying fluid will shunt the responses being recorded by population electrodes. Visualization is done using nonwater immersion objectives. The electrodes used are similar to patch clamp electrodes except that they are just inserted into the region of interest in the extracellular space. Population responses are observed as changes in the multicellular activity around the tip of the electrode, and sophisticated analysis programs, such as MatLab software (The MathWorks, Natick, MA), need to be used. Plots of the event-related spectral perturbation (ERSP) for each population response can be generated with the EEGLAB MatLab Toolbox. These analyses generate power spectra for continuous points in time, for example, during and after application of an agent or washout. These graphs show plot frequency of activity over time, and the amplitude of the frequency shown is color-coded such that background (control) appears light green, and higher amplitudes appear progressively more yellow, then red. For example, cholinergic input into the PPN can be tested using different concentrations of CAR. Application of different concentrations of CAR to the PPN reveals that rhythmic oscillations can be induced by CAR in a dose-dependent manner. For example, CAR induces peaks of activity at theta and gamma band, with the increases in the gamma range being significantly higher (Figure 6.2). Significantly, when modafinil is applied, the agent by itself does not produce a specific response, but when CAR is reapplied after 20 minutes of exposure to modafinil, the response to CAR is amplified. The increased coherence enabled by modafinil is evident in the ERSPs generated from the population responses. This suggests that modafinil-induced increases in electrical coupling may amplify the responses of PPN neurons to transmitter inputs. In general, these results suggest that (a) gamma band activity appears to be part of the intrinsic membrane properties of PPN neurons, (b) the population as a whole generates gamma band activity under the influence of specific transmitters, and (c) modafinil appears to amplify the response to some transmitters. These studies as a whole allow extrapolation of results from slices to predict responses in vivo in whole animals and humans, a powerful set of translational research tools.

PRECONSCIOUS AWARENESS

What is the role of gamma band activity in the RAS? People often act in order to meet desired goals, and feel that conscious will is the cause of their behavior. Scientific research suggests otherwise. Under some conditions, actions are initiated even though we are unconscious of the goal. Libet

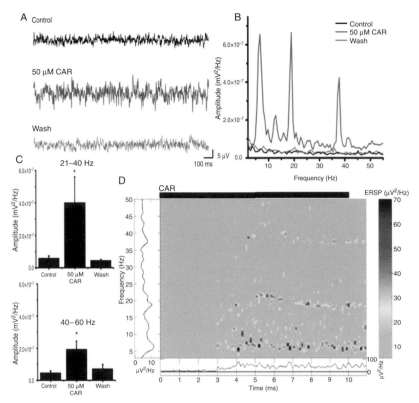

Figure 6.2   Carbachol (CAR) application increased activity at theta, low, and mid gamma frequencies. (A) One sec sample recording before (black), during (red), and following (brown) application of CAR (30 μM). (B) Power spectrum of 20-second record- ings, including the one sec shown in (A). Specific peaks were observed in the theta, low, and mid gamma ranges. (C) Amplitude of the response in four slices was quantified and a significant increase in activity in the low (upper graph) and medium gamma range (lower graph) was observed (***$p < 0.001$, **$p < 0.01$, *$p < 0.05$). (D) Graph of event- related spectral perturbations (ERSPs) using ($n = 10$) 20-second recordings during CAR application. The effect of CAR started at minute 3, with a peak effect after 5 minutes. During the peak effect, CAR induced oscillations at specific frequencies in the theta, low gamma, and medium gamma ranges. (For color details, please see the color plate section.)

was the first to show that when people consciously set a goal to engage in a behavior, their conscious will to act starts out unconsciously [7]. Libet recorded the Readiness Potential (RP), a negative DC shift present long before the execution of a voluntary movement, in people asked to move voluntarily, and were also asked to subjectively time the will to move and the subjective timing of the onset of movement. (Note: The RP is maximal over the vertex, the same region described in the preceding text where the P50 potential [2] and equivalent magnetic M50 response [8] are maximal, and where PPN deep brain stimulation produces the greatest changes in cortical blood flow [9].) The initial and later phases of the RP preceded the consciously determined will to move by hundreds of milliseconds. The authors concluded that cerebral initiation of spontaneous, freely voluntary acts could begin unconsciously, before there is any subjective awareness that a decision to act was initiated cerebrally. Even simple movements appear to be generated subconsciously, and the conscious sense of volition comes later [10]. This review describes the details of studies showing that voluntary movements can be triggered with stimuli that are not perceived, that movement may well occur prior to the apparent planning of the movement, and that not only the sense of willing the movement, but also the sense of the movement having occurred, happens before the actual movement [10].

Is there a mechanism, perhaps based on intrinsic oscillatory activity, that generates a similar process but at subcortical levels? Gamma band activity has been reported in the hippocampus and cerebellum. Now, three nuclei that are part of the RAS all exhibit electrical coupling, providing a novel mechanism for sleep-wake control based on coherence driven by electrical coupling [3,5,6]. Moreover, virtually ALL neurons in these nuclei, regardless of cell or transmitter type, exhibit gamma band activity generated by intrinsic membrane properties. Regardless of depolarizing level or input, these cells are "pegged" to fire at gamma band frequency (30 60 Hz) [3,5,6]. This is a very unique property. Taken together, these results suggest that a similar mechanism to that in the cortex for achieving temporal coherence at high frequencies is present in the PPN, and perhaps its subcortical targets such as the Pf and SubCD nuclei. We suggested that gamma band activity generated in the PPN may help stabilize coherence related to arousal, providing a stable activation state during waking and paradoxical sleep [6]. Our overall hypothesis here is that sensory input will induce gamma band activity in the RAS that could participate in preconscious awareness. The RAS seems the ideal site for sub or preconscious awareness since it is phylogenetically conserved, modulates sleep/wake cycles, the startle response, and fight-or-flight responses that include changes in muscle tone and locomotion.

The clinical implications of these findings are only now being addressed, and they could open the way for a number of clinical applications and interventions based on the fact that some cells in the RAS are electrically coupled, and many more cells in the RAS can fire at gamma band frequencies. The use of the vertex-recorded P13 potential in the freely moving rat, and the human P50 potential can both be used to address this newly discovered mechanism.

MAGNETOENCEPHALOGRAPHY, THE CADILLAC OF HUMAN ELECTROPHYSIOLOGY

Perhaps the most useful method for assessing brain activity in real time is with the use of magnetoencephalography (MEG). In the future, this technology may be as common as the EEG; however, lack of knowledge and the high cost of the technology have slowed its dissemination. If a translational neuroscience program is to thrive, an MEG may be an absolute, but expensive, necessity. MEG and EEG are two complementary techniques that measure the magnetic induction outside the head and the scalp of the electric potentials produced by electrical activity in neural assemblies. They directly measure brain activity in the millisecond range, that is, in real time, and current forms of analysis allow spatial localization in the 1–2 mm range. Moreover, a number of source localization methods have been developed to coalesce functional MEG recordings with anatomical MRI data. The MEG measures the flow of postsynaptic currents in the dendrites of cortical neurons. Typical neuromagnetic signals are in the order of 50–500 femtoTesla (minute magnetic power) in amplitude and require the activation of 10,000–100,000 neurons in time and space, that is, intracellular currents must be aligned in space (the fact that the cortex is a laminar structure allows such alignment) and activated around the same time to permit minimal cancellation and maximal summation of the magnetic field. However, even the strongest responses generated by the brain are orders of magnitude weaker than ambient magnetic signals such as the earth's magnetic field, moving vehicles, power lines, and the human heart.

Therefore, the MEG requires an extremely sensitive system, Superconducting Quantum Interference Devices (SQUIDs), which are low temperature amplifiers able to detect minute changes in the magnetic flux through magnetometer coils in a superconducting environment. The latest arrays include over 300 sensors immersed in a Dewar cooled with liquid helium. The array of SQUID magnetometers or gradiometers arranged outside the head act as induction coils that, due to their superconductive properties, can adequately detect the magnetic field associated with currents in cortical neurons. Appropriate noise cancellation methods include second and third order gradiometers that cancel magnetic fields generated by distant sources, and shielded rooms that divert magnetic noise away from the sensor array. High-frequency perturbations such as radiofrequency waves are easily attenuated in a shielded room made of successive layers of mu-metal, copper, and aluminum. Low-frequency artifacts generated by vehicles, elevators, and other moving objects are attenuated by the use of gradiometers as sensing units. The signals generated are then used to analyze cortical dynamics using event-related field calculations to measure responses time locked to a stimulus, spectrotemporal change quantification to analyze signals in the frequency domain, and principal component and independent component analyses to detect signal separation.

The major attraction of the MEG is that, while the EEG is extremely sensitive to the effects of secondary or volume currents, MEG is more sensitive to the primary current sources in the brain. The ability of MEG to detect not only the source of seizures in the brain, but also to localize the initial ictal event, has become the method of choice for mapping epilepsy surgery, to the point that spontaneous recordings, evoked recordings, and functional mapping are now reimbursed by insurers. In fact, much of the maintenance of a MEG can come from such reimbursements.

Spontaneous MEG activity can provide significant information concerning global functional brain states in normal individuals and in certain neurological and psychiatric patients. To quantify the oscillatory activity of the brain, the averaged magnetic power spectrum is calculated. This gives a measure of the amplitude of the magnetic signal at each frequency and can be used to distinguish normal and abnormal brain activity. The average of the mean power spectra for a set of normal awake individuals at rest, and for a set of awake resting patients with, for example, Parkinson's disease (PD) show that the control plot is characterized by an alpha rhythm (10–12 Hz) peaking at 10 Hz, while the power in PD patients is shifted to lower frequency in the theta range (4–8 Hz). Patient populations with such a shift, in which the low frequency band is increased and alpha band activity is decreased, are referred to as having thalamocortical dysrhythmia (TCD). TCD patients also show a large power correlation across a wide span of frequencies, whereas normal subjects do not show much power across all frequencies (this is determined by plotting the average power of all MEG channels against itself). The cellular mechanisms behind this effect have been proposed to arise from thalamocortical slowing due to decreased activation or overinhibition of the thalamus that leads to excessive bursting (rather than tonic) activity. Regardless of the exact mechanism, a number of other disorders show a similar increase in MEG power in the theta band, and the associated increase in power correlation within the theta and between the theta and the beta/gamma bands [11].

Considerable evidence has been published to support the idea that thalamocortical resonance, as determined using the MEG, is not only a prerequisite for cognition, but that its perturbation (i.e., TCD) can underlie a variety of neurological and psychiatric disorders. Essentially, this slowing is thought to perturb normal sensation, providing misinformation to the central nervous system (CNS). Confirmatory evidence using single cell recordings from excessively bursting neurons in the intralaminar thalamus of humans has been reported for PD, tinnitus, chronic pain, psychosis, anxiety disorder/obsessive compulsive disorder, epilepsy, dystonia, and spasticity patients [11]. Convincing data demonstrate that electrolytic lesion of abnormally firing cells in these patients reduced or resolved the symptoms in most patients [12]. These lesions led to a normalization of MEG power spectra such that, in patients with symptom relief, TCD was eliminated and spontaneous alpha band power returned. The key to improving clinical outcome is to determine if patients with such disorders indeed have TCD. If they do, then thalamocortical rhythms are evidently involved, but if they do not have TCD, then nonthalamic disturbances are suspected. For example, if a chronic pain patient has TCD, he would not be a candidate for implanting a spinal transcutaneous electrical nerve stimulation (TENS) unit for alleviation of pain (because, probably, the pain is neurogenic or being "generated" in the thalamus, not in the spinal cord), but if he does not have TCD, the pain may indeed be of spinal origin and a TENS unit would have a better chance of producing a salutary effect.

Spontaneous MEG recordings can be carried out to determine power spectra as an index of coherence, and also to determine the presence of TCD in subjects across a number of conditions. This may allow the identification of subpopulations of patients with each condition with and without TCD. The use of evoked responses will also provide valuable information, especially using a paired stimulus paradigm, in which the M50 response (the magnetic equivalent of the P50 potential [8]) to the first stimulus provides a measure of level of arousal (decreased arousal is present in narcolepsy, autism, and some AD patients). The response to the second stimulus, specifically the ratio of the two responses, provides a measure of habituation (decreased habituation is present in schizophrenia, posttraumatic stress disorder (PTSD), depression, some AD patients, Huntington's disease, and PD patients). Go-no go responses present additional discriminatory opportunities in disorders of volition and movement, for example, PD, dystonia, spasticity, and so on. Reaction time, provided by the go response is also the prototypical measure of attention, allowing one to quantitatively assess this process [8].

REFERENCES

1. Kezunovic K, Simon C, Hyde J, Smith K, Beck P, Odle A, Garcia-Rill E. (2010) Translational studies on sleep-wake control. Transl Neurosci 1, 2–8.
2. Garcia-Rill E, Skinner RD. (2001) The sleep state-dependent P50 midlatency auditory evoked potential. In: Lee-Chiong TL, Carskadon MA, Sateia MJ, eds. Sleep Medicine. Philadelphia: Hanley & Belfus, pp. 697–704.
3. Garcia-Rill E, Heister DS, Ye M, Charlesworth A, Hayar A. (2007) Electrical coupling: novel mechanism for sleep-wake control. Sleep 30, 1405–1414.
4. Urbano FJ, Leznik E, Llinas R. (2007) Modafinil enhances thalamocortical activity by increasing neuronal electrotonic coupling. Proc Natl Acad Sci USA 104, 12554–12559.
5. Beck P, Odle A, Wallace-Huitt T, Skinner RD, Garcia-Rill E. (2008) Modafinil increases arousal determined by P13 potential amplitude: an effect blocked by gap junction antagonists. Sleep 31, 1647–1654.
6. Kezunovic N, Urbano FJ, Simon C, Hyde J, Smith K, Garcia-Rill E. (2011) Mechanism behind gamma band activity in the pedunculopontine nucleus (PPN). Eur J Neurosci 34, 404–415.
7. Libet B, Gleason CA, Wright EW, Pearl DK. (1983) Time of conscious intention to act in relation to onset of cerebral activity (readiness-potential). The unconscious initiation of a freely voluntary act. Brain 106, 623–642.

8. Garcia-Rill E, Moran K, Garcia J, Findley WM, Walton K, Strotman B, Llinas R. (2008) Magnetic sources of the M50 response are localized to frontal cortex. Clin Neurophysiol 119, 388–398.

9. Ballanger B, Lozano AM, Moro E, van Eimeren T, Hamani C, Chen R, Cilia R, Houle S, Poon YY, Lang AE, Strafella AP. (2009) Cerebral blood flow changes induced by pedunculopontine nucleus stimulation in patients with advanced Parkinson's disease: a [(15)O] H2O PET study. Human Brain Mapp 30, 3901–3909.

10. Hallett M. (2007) Volitional control of movement: the physiology of free will. Clin Neurophysiol 118, 1179–1192.

11. Llinas R, Ribary U, Jeanmonod D, Cancro R, Kronberg E, Schulman J, Zonenshayn M, Magnin M, Morel A, Siegmund M. (2001) Thalamocortical dysrhythmia I. Functional and imaging aspects. Thal Relat Syst 1, 237–244.

12. Jeanmonod D, Magnin M, Morel A, Siegemund M, Cancro A, Lanz M, Llinás R, Ribary U, Kronberg E, Schulman J, Zonenshayn M. (2001) Thalamocortical dysrhythmia II. Clinical and surgical aspects. Thal Relat Syst 1, 245–254.

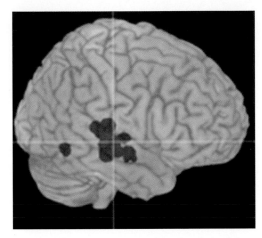

Figure 4.2   Region of interest plot. A circular "region of interest" denotes the location of each treatment site. A subtraction procedure (in MRICroN) revealed sites common to participants who responded (i.e., BA 22, designated by the crosshair) but not to nonresponders.

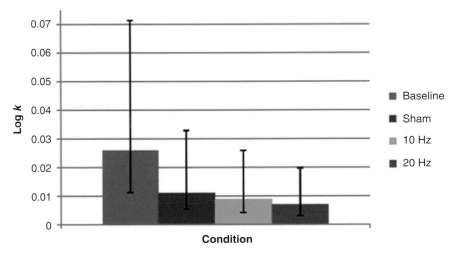

Figure 4.3   Delay discounting graphs. Discounting rate (k) by condition calculated using a hyperbolic-delay equation $v_d = V/(1 + kd)$, where v_d is the discounted value of a delayed reward, V is the objective value of the delayed reward, k is an empirically derived constant proportional to the degree of delay discounting, and d is delay duration. Main effect of condition $p = 0.02$; post hoc tests: baseline/10 Hz $p = 0.03$; baseline/20 Hz $p = 0.005$.

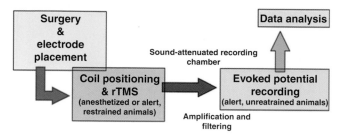

Figure 4.4 Protocol for TMS in animals. Diagram of the experimental protocol for TMS in animals.

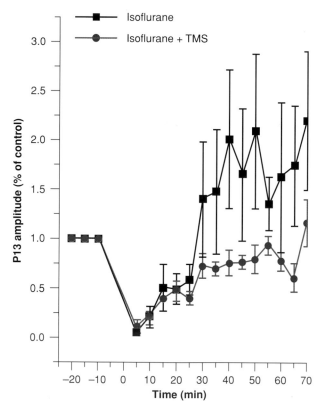

Figure 4.5 Effects of anesthesia and TMS on the P13 potential. Representative measurements of the amplitude of the conditioning response exposure to isoflurane anesthesia with and without rTMS.

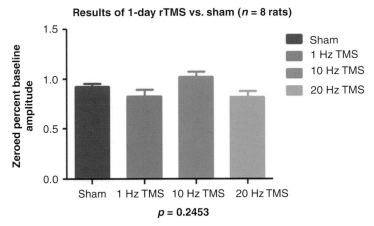

Figure 4.6 Effect of single-session rTMS on P13 potential amplitude. Note that TMS did not induce significant changes when applied at 1 Hz, 10 Hz, or 20 Hz, suggesting that TMS by itself does not alter the acute manifestation of the P13 potential. This establishes single-session TMS as a method that does not alter arousal, opening its use as a method to reduce or alter treatments that increase or decrease arousal levels.

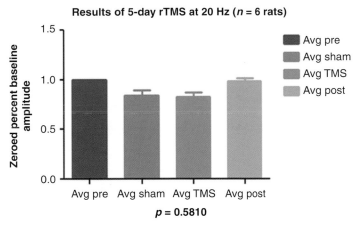

Figure 4.7 Effect of multiple session rTMS on P13 potential amplitude. Treatment with TMS similar to that used in humans (five daily rTMS sessions) failed to alter P13 potential amplitude in the rat compared with pre-TMS control or sham stimulation. In addition, P13 potential amplitude was not affected following rTMS, suggesting that multiple session TMS does not alter arousal, opening its use as a method to reduce or alter treatments that increase or decrease arousal levels.

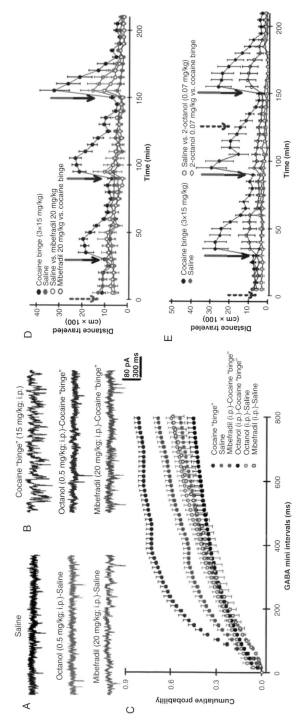

Figure 5.1   Cocaine-induced involvement of *T*-type calcium channels in thalamocortical GABAergic transmission. Coadministration of *T*-type calcium channel blockers prevented cocaine-mediated enhancement of GABAergic transmission onto VB neurons in vivo. Representative GABAergic mini currents in VB neurons recorded from mice injected with saline ((A) without and with previous in vivo i.p. injections of 2-octanol 0.5 mg/kg or mibefradil 20 mg/kg) or cocaine ((B) 3 × 15 mg/kg, 1 hour apart and with 2-octanol 0.5 mg/kg and mibefradil 20 mg/kg). (C) Average cumulative probability plots of GABAergic mini interevent intervals recorded in VB neurons from mice injected with all combinations showed in (A) and (B). Note how GABAergic mini interevent intervals were significantly affected by in vivo administration of *T*-type calcium blockers 2-octanol and mibefradil (see the text). (D) Mibefradil reduced cocaine-induced hyperlocomotion. Plot showing the average distance traveled (in cm × 100) by mice i.p.-injected with saline (gray-filled circles), cocaine (red-filled circles), saline pretreated with mibefradil (empty gray circles) and cocaine pretreated with mibefradil (empty green circles). (E) Same as (D), for 2-octanol (0.07 mg/kg).

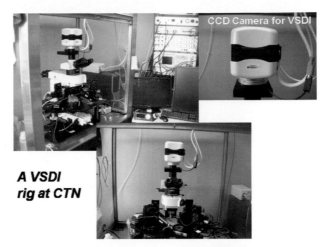

Figure 5.2 Photomicrographs showing voltage-sensitive dye imaging (VSDI) and patch clamp rig. Upper left image shows low-magnification photograph of the voltage sensitive dye rig. Upper right image shows detailed photograph of the Evolve camera used for VSDI recordings. Middle lower photograph shows micromanipulator arrangement and interface chamber used for VSDI experiments located on top of a Gibraltar stage in combination with an upright microscope.

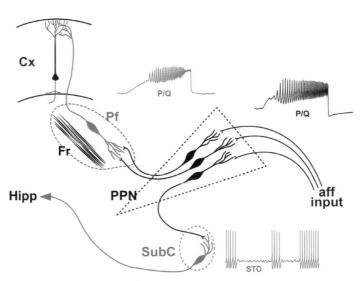

Figure 6.1 Gamma band activity in the reticular activating system (RAS). Wiring diagram of RAS nuclei manifesting gamma band activity and the mechanisms behind these oscillations. Afferent input that originates from collateral activation of the RAS by sensory systems activates the dendrites of pedunculopontine nucleus (PPN) neurons. The presence of P/Q- and N-type calcium channels in the dendrites set off oscillations at gamma band that influence firing frequency. The output of the PPN descends to the subcoeruleus (SubC), presumably activating these neurons that have sodium-dependent subthreshold oscillations. These cells in turn influence downstream systems involved in the atonia of REM sleep, and ascending systems that may participate in the consolidation of memories such as the hippocampus (Hipp). The output of the PPN also ascends to the intralaminar thalamus, especially the parafascicular (Pf) nucleus, activating its dendrites to oscillate at gamma frequency via P/Q- and N-type calcium channels. These cells in turn project to the cortex, particularly to upper cortical layers where the nonspecific thalamic inputs terminate, to activate cortical neurons. Once cortical, hippocampal, and cerebellar cells are activated, the generation and maintenance of gamma band activity in the brain can more easily be maintained.

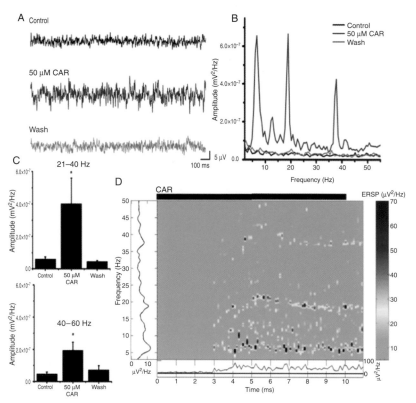

Figure 6.2 Carbachol (CAR) application increased activity at theta, low, and mid gamma frequencies. (A) One sec sample recording before (black), during (red), and following (brown) application of CAR (30 μM). (B) Power spectrum of 20-second recordings, including the one sec shown in (A). Specific peaks were observed in the theta, low, and mid gamma ranges. (C) Amplitude of the response in four slices was quantified and a significant increase in activity in the low (upper graph) and medium gamma range (lower graph) was observed (***$p < 0.001$, **$p < 0.01$, *$p < 0.05$). (D) Graph of event-related spectral perturbations (ERSPs) using ($n = 10$) 20-second recordings during CAR application. The effect of CAR started at minute 3, with a peak effect after 5 minutes. During the peak effect, CAR induced oscillations at specific frequencies in the theta, low gamma, and medium gamma ranges.

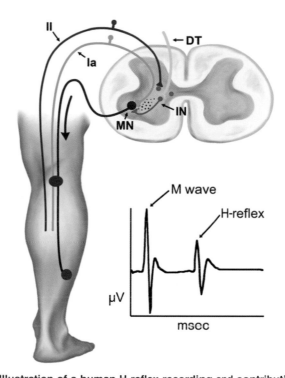

Figure 7.1 Illustration of a human H-reflex recording and contributing pathways and a representation of an H-reflex recording in the rat. A stimulus delivered to the popliteal fossa (large black oval, stimulating electrode) first produces an orthodromic (descending dark-blue pathway) volley recorded over the soleus muscle (small black circle, recording electrode), as the initial motor (M wave) response. The same stimulus will activate ascending Ia fibers (green pathway) antidromically that results in a monosynaptic connection with the MN. This activation induces a response that descends (dark-blue pathway) and is recorded over the soleus muscle in the human as the longer latency H-reflex. Mechanisms that have been proposed to contribute to spasticity include (a) loss of presynaptic inhibition of group Ia and II afferent (red pathway) fibers due to loss of descending inhibition from DTs (light-blue pathway), (b) intrinsic changes of the MN, (c) upregulation of postsynaptic receptors, and (d) terminal sprouting. The present results also suggest that changes in electrical coupling in the area of the interneurons (IN, medium-blue pathway) occur after SCI. Interventions outlined in the text include oral modafinil that might influence changes in electrical coupling at the level of the interneurons and MN, passive exercise resulting in possible changes to the MN, and L-dopa, which has been suggested to influence the group II afferent pathways. DT, descending tract; IN, inhibitory interneuron; MN, motoneuron; Ia, group Ia afferent fibers; II, group II afferent fibers; small dots in the medial ventral spinal cord represent Renshaw cells; SCI, spinal cord injury. (Reproduced by permission from Translational Neurosci 2010, 1(2), 161.)

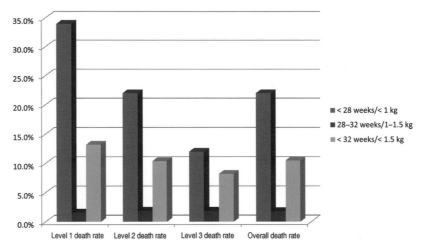

Figure 8.1 Mortality rate. Note the increased mortality rate in neonates <1 kg in the lower level nurseries compared with the level 3 nursery. *p <0.001 for babies <1000 g and/or <28 weeks in level 3 nurseries compared with level 1 or 2 nurseries.

7 Translational Research on Spinal Cord Injury

Charlotte Yates and Kevin Garrison

The symptoms of spinal cord injury (SCI) are devastating, including, among others, loss of locomotor control, muscle atrophy, and hyperreflexia/spasticity. Most basic research has been directed at compensating for the deficits produced by approaches aimed at regenerating the pathways involved. However, the clinical application of regenerative therapies is far in the future. Our approach has been to develop therapeutic avenues that can be developed to help the patient with a SCI now rather than later. For example, we know that the spinal cord has pattern generators that contain the preprogrammed sequence of flexion-extension alternation for each limb [1]. We reasoned that SCI induced a regression to a neonatal state in which the spinal cord was devoid of descending supraspinal input. What parameters of stimulation were needed to elicit locomotion in the neonatal spinal cord (before supraspinal input was established), so that we might use those parameters to determine if the spinal cord can be driven by such stimuli after SCI? We undertook the development of the in vitro brainstem spinal cord preparation and were the first to demonstrate electrical- and chemically induced locomotion in the 0–4-day-old brainstem-spinal cord of the rat [2]. We then used the same parameters of stimulation (long duration, low-frequency pulses) in the neonate rat to induce locomotion following epidural stimulation in the acutely spinalized adult cat [3]. We then patented a method and device for epidural stimulation of the spinal cord to induce locomotion in the human [4], and helped others demonstrate that the method could be used to induce locomotion in human SCI victims [5]. Another approach was to use passive exercise to attempt to slow or combat the muscle atrophy induced by SCI, and we found that passive cycling exercise in the rat could restore muscle mass after 90 days of daily cycling [6], although the amount of time needed in the human would be more in the order of 6–9 months and have not been able to establish sufficient compliance. However, passive exercise has proven

Translational Neuroscience: A Guide to a Successful Program, First Edition. Edited by Edgar Garcia-Rill.
© 2012 John Wiley & Sons, Inc. Published 2012 by John Wiley & Sons, Inc.

to be beneficial in the restoration of normal reflexes after SCI in rats and humans [7,8]. In this chapter, we will discuss interventions that have been explored to address two symptoms that result from SCI, hyperreflexia and spasticity, which can contribute to significant functional limitations.

ELECTROPHYSIOLOGICAL APPROACH: H-REFLEX FREQUENCY-DEPENDENT DEPRESSION

Hyperreflexia is a component of spasticity and develops over time in both the human and animal following SCI [9,10]. We used the H-reflex to quantify hyperreflexia in both the patient with SCI and the complete transection model of SCI in the rat. The H-reflex is a compound electromyographic (EMG) response that can be recorded from the muscle following activation of motor neurons via muscle afferents that are stimulated by applying an electrical current to the nerve (Figure 7.1). The H-reflex is rate sensitive in spinally intact individuals and demonstrates depressed amplitude, due to marked habituation, once stimulus frequencies reach or exceed 1 Hz [1–3,5–8,11,12]. In patients with SCI or animals with chronic SCI, frequency-dependent depression (FDD) of the H-reflex is markedly decreased [10]. Thus, FDD has been used by many investigators as a quantitative measure of hyperreflexia.

Original H-reflex recordings [13] involved a terminal procedure done under ketamine anesthesia. This technique allowed direct visualization and stimulation of the tibial nerve with a hook electrode, and intramuscular recording by fine wire inserted in the interosseous muscle of the hind paw. While these terminal recordings provided a great amount of control, we desired to have a technique that would more closely mimic the conditions for the human H-reflex recordings and to avoid the effects of anesthesia on the reflex. A percutaneous approach was developed that utilized two needle electrodes that were inserted under the skin near the tibial nerve with recording done by dry gel electrodes placed on the skin of the hind paw. After refinement, this new technique proved to be highly correlated with the terminal procedure and provided the added benefit of allowing for longitudinal recordings in the same animal [14].

Thompson [15] found a delayed onset of hyperreflexia in the contusion animal model of SCI when there was no significant difference between control animals and animals with a contusion SCI measured 6 days after injury. These authors reported a significant decrease in FDD of the monosynaptic reflex at 28 and 60 days postcontusion. That is, there was a delay between the injury and the onset of hyperreflexia. The time course of development of hyperreflexia was similar in the complete transection model of SCI and a decrease in FDD occurred between 7 and 14 days posttransection and changes plateaued after 30 days following transection [16]. Schindler-Ivens

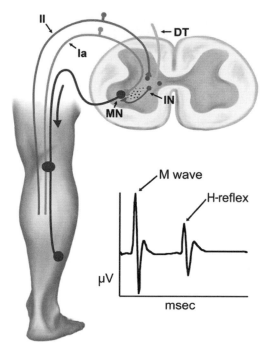

Figure 7.1 Illustration of a human H-reflex recording and contributing pathways and a representation of an H-reflex recording in the rat. A stimulus delivered to the popliteal fossa (large black oval, stimulating electrode) first produces an orthodromic (descending dark-blue pathway) volley recorded over the soleus muscle (small black circle, recording electrode), as the initial motor (M wave) response. The same stimulus will activate ascending Ia fibers (green pathway) antidromically that results in a monosynaptic connection with the MN. This activation induces a response that descends (dark-blue pathway) and is recorded over the soleus muscle in the human as the longer latency H-reflex. Mechanisms that have been proposed to contribute to spasticity include (a) loss of presynaptic inhibition of group Ia and II afferent (red pathway) fibers due to loss of descending inhibition from DTs (light-blue pathway), (b) intrinsic changes of the MN, (c) upregulation of postsynaptic receptors, and (d) terminal sprouting. The present results also suggest that changes in electrical coupling in the area of the interneurons (IN, medium-blue pathway) occur after SCI. Interventions outlined in the text include oral modafinil that might influence changes in electrical coupling at the level of the interneurons and MN, passive exercise resulting in possible changes to the MN, and L-dopa, which has been suggested to influence the group II afferent pathways. DT, descending tract; IN, inhibitory interneuron; MN, motoneuron; Ia, group Ia afferent fibers; II, group II afferent fibers; small dots in the medial ventral spinal cord represent Renshaw cells; SCI, spinal cord injury. (Reproduced by permission from Yates C, Garrison MK, Reese NB, Garcia-Rill E. (2010) Therapeutic approaches for spinal cord Injury induced spasticity. Translational Neurosci 1, 160–169.) (For color details, please see the color plate section.)

and Shields [10] investigated the time course of the development of hyperreflexia in a patient with a SCI and reported FDD changes occurred between 6–18 weeks after injury, with continued changes occurring until 44 weeks postinjury. That is, the time course of the onset in the human was longer than in the rat.

While the H-reflex FDD has provided valuable insight into changes in reflex activity following SCI, it fails to capture the full complexity of the spastic motor behaviors that are often present following injury. Previous reviews [17] have discussed the possible pathophysiology of spasticity involving spinal networks beyond the simple monosynaptic stretch reflex. These mechanisms include cellular changes that manifest plateau potentials, alteration in the normal disynaptic inhibition, and recent exploration of changes in gap junctions between spinal neurons [18]. To date, there is no gold standard for the quantification of spasticity, but we felt a combined approach of adding biomechanical measures to the electrophysiological measures would provide a more complete picture of pathological reflexes [19].

BIOMECHANICAL APPROACH: WINDUP OF THE STRETCH REFLEX

Spasticity is defined as a velocity-dependent increase in resistance to muscle stretch and its onset in humans is delayed following SCI. The rat model of SCI has also been shown to demonstrate this velocity-dependent increase in resistance (torque) and EMG activity [15]. Clinical measures of spasticity include the Ashworth test but it has been shown to have low interrater reliability due in part to the difficulty of distinguishing passive muscle tension from true velocity-dependent changes in resistance to movement. Laboratory approaches range from instrumented pendulum drop tests to more complex powered devices that measure the response to imposed sinusoidal perturbations [20]. One laboratory approach that has been used to assess spasticity in humans is based on the phenomenon of temporal facilitation or windup of stretch reflexes [21]. This windup effect is attributed to intracellular plateau potentials that result in sustained depolarization in motoneurons (MN). The sustained activity is due to the presence of persistent inward currents (PICs) that are associated with the onset of spasticity in animals [22]. Notably, PICs are dependent on neuromodulation from the brainstem, which is rendered ineffective on spinal cord cells in SCI. However, recent work provides evidence for the presence of constitutively activated 5-HT receptors in spinal MN in chronic in vivo preparations [23]. As a tool to study spasticity, the stretch reflex windup protocol offers a noninvasive measure with valuable insight into the mechanism behind spasticity and has the benefit of providing a means to normalize the responses (peak/initial) to allow longitudinal and intersubject comparisons. While spinal intact controls fail to demonstrate temporal facilitation in response to repeated stretches, patients with SCI show a windup of the torque and EMG response to repeated stretches at intervals less than 1 second. In a bedside-to-bench approach, we decided to examine if the complete transection model of rat SCI also demonstrates temporal facilitation of the stretch reflex.

A purpose-built actuator was constructed to provide controlled perturbations to the ankle while recording reactive torque of the plantar flexor muscles. Ten high velocity stretches were applied at frequencies of 1, 2, and 4 Hz on a weekly basis beginning 1-week posttransection. As hypothesized, windup was present in the animal model but the onset was found to be delayed in comparison to the onset of H-reflex FDD as discussed earlier. Although stretch reflexes were present as early as 1-week posttransection, windup of the torque and EMG response to repeated stretch did not appear until 42-days posttransection [24]. This confirmed that the two measures are not redundant but provide a multifaceted insight into different mechanisms associated with the complex neural plasticity following SCI. One of the drawbacks of this approach is that efforts to create a control group in the animal model are stymied by the fact that repeated plantar flexion stretches in a spinally intact rat tends to produce avoidance behavior and voluntary firing of the hind limb muscles that mask any reflex responses (or lack thereof). As a result, we had to refer to findings from intact humans who do not demonstrate windup of the stretch reflex.

INTERVENTIONS: PASSIVE EXERCISE

We investigated the use of a motorized bicycle exercise trainer (MBET) to provide passive exercise to normalize hyperreflexia and/or spasticity. We have also investigated optimal parameters for cycling training that are required for adult rats with complete SCIs as well as training for patients with a classification of ASIA A or B (complete lack of motor control). The initial work examined if passive exercise training would alter FDD of the H-reflex and/or the SR in the animal model, and then the focus shifted to ideal training regimens. We were also interested in the training effects to modulate the spinal cord circuitry in the acute phase of injury (prior to the onset of hyperreflexia) compared with the chronic phase of injury (after hyperreflexia has been established). We questioned whether the effects we were observing would be maintained if cessation of training were to occur. Finally, we examined the effects of passive training in patients with SCI.

As previously mentioned, the onset of hyperreflexia and spasticity do not have an identical time course. We anticipated then that the effects of passive training might be different for these two outcome measures. Initial publications [8,13] reported that passive exercise training initiated in the acute phase of injury (prior to onset of hyperreflexia) could restore FDD of spinal reflexes in a time-dependent manner. The training time of 30 days with a training schedule of 1 hour a day, 5 days a week resulted in a statistically significant difference ($p < 0.05$) for all frequencies tested compared with the transected animals that had not been trained. This finding progressed to a series of experiments to determine the optimal training required for different phases of injury.

Figure 7.2 illustrates the onset of hyperreflexia that is delayed after injury and the changes to the H-reflex FDD plateaus at 30-days posttransection, Figure 7.2 also illustrates the impact of the duration of training during different phases of injury. A training program of passive exercise training (initiated prior to hyperreflexia being established) required 30 days of training for 1 hour a day, 5 times per week. However, if the passive exercise was initiated in the chronic stage of injury (after hyperreflexia was established), the training program required 60 days of training at the 1 hour per day, 5 times per week schedule. This result was consistent with

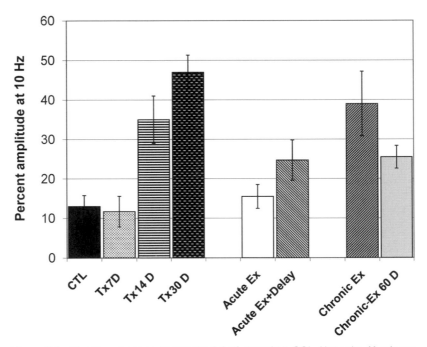

Figure 7.2   H-reflex changes in the model of complete SCI. Along the X-axis represents groups of animals and the Y-axis represents the average amplitude of the H-reflex at 10 Hz. Compared to CTL, the Tx14D group is significantly different at $p < 0.05$ and the Tx30D group is significantly different at $p < 0.01$. The next set of groups involved exercise. Acute Ex is equal to Tx + MBET 30 days, which differed from the Tx only group at $p < 0.01$. Acute Ex + Delay is equal to Tx +MBET 30 days and then cessation of exercise. This group was able to maintain H-reflex changes that differed from the Tx only group at $p < 0.05$. The final section of the graph represents exercise that is initiated after hyperreflexia is established. Chronic-Ex is equal to Tx, no exercise for 30 days then MBET 30 days. The Chronic-Ex was not statistically different that the Tx only group. Chronic-Ex 60 is equal to Tx and no exercise 30 days then MBET 60 days. The Ch-Ex 60D is significantly different that the Tx only group at $p < 0.01$. CTL, control group of intact animals; Tx7D, Tx and H-reflex recorded after 7-days postinjury; Tx14D, Tx and H-reflex recorded after 14 days postinjury; Tx30D, Tx and H-reflex recorded after 30 days postinjury.

training effects observed in the contusion model of SCI [25]. In summary, twice the duration of exercise was required to show modulation of the spinal circuitry when training was initiated in the chronic phase of injury compared to the acute phase.

Later investigations of the exercise effect on the stretch reflex had mixed results. Similar to the H-reflex measure, when passive exercise was initiated prior to the onset of SR windup, 30 days of training was sufficient for the prevention of SR windup (Figure 7.3). Further study is needed to examine the necessary dosage of passive exercise when initiated after 42 days (chronic stage) when the presence of SR windup has been established. These data would provide information on the optimal exercise parameters that could be translated to individuals with chronic SCI who would be likely candidates for a MBET program.

A motorized bicycle training program was studied in a patient with SCI when initiated in the chronic phase of injury, 1 year after SCI [7]. This patient demonstrated that passive exercise could lead to habituation of the H-reflex after 8–10 weeks of 1 hour a day, 5 times per week training

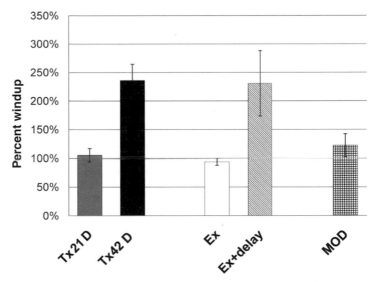

Figure 7.3 Stretch Reflex changes in the model of complete SCI. The X-axis denotes the various groups of animals and the Y-axis represents the mean ($\pm$SE) peak plantarflexion torque response to repeated stretches as a percent of the first stretch (%windup). Groups are compared to Tx42D when windup of the SR emerges. Tx21D was significantly different ($p < 0.01$), demonstrating a delayed onset as compared to the H-reflex. Ex and MOD interventions demonstrated a normalization effect on windup with significance difference from Tx42D ($p < 0.01$). Ex+delay animals failed to retain the training effects and the percent windup was no different than Tx42D ($p > 0.1$). Tx21D, 21 days post-Tx; Tx42D, 42 days post-Tx; Ex, Tx then MBET for 30 days; Ex+Delay, Tx then MBET for 30 days followed by 28 days without exercise; MOD, Tx then MOD administration for 30 days.

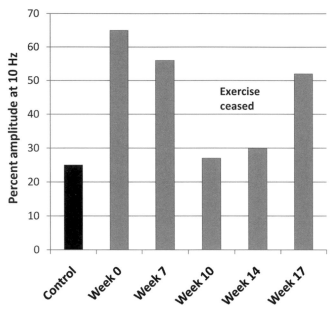

Figure 7.4   H-reflex changes in the patient with SCI. The effect of MBET on the H-reflex FDD at 10 Hz for a patient with SCI. Habituation of the H-reflex was measured over the course of 13 weeks of MBET sessions (1 hour per day, 5x per week) in a patient with a chronic SCI (ASIA B) and established hyperreflexia and spasticity. Control values were based upon mean H-reflex FDD in 16 spinally intact individuals and were used for statistical comparisons. The average values of the H-reflex amplitudes are significantly different ($p < 0.01$) when comparing weeks 1–6 to weeks 10–15. As indicated by the arrow, cessation of MBET occurred at 13 weeks. By week 17, the habituation of the H-reflex was no longer present. MBET, motorized bicycle exercise trainer; FDD, frequency-dependent depression; SCI, spinal cord injury.

(Figure 7.4). MBET in a tandem setup has been shown to be effective in reducing hyperreflexia in patients with an incomplete SCI [26]. Further research is indicated to determine the effects of cycling training when initiated in the acute stages of injury and effects of training on spasticity in addition to the effects on hyperreflexia.

What if cessation of training occurs? Cessation of training has revealed different effects depending on whether the exercise training was initiated in the acute phase of injury versus the chronic phase of injury in the animal model and the patient with a SCI. The modulation of the FDD of the H-reflex was maintained in the animal model of SCI (Figure 7.2) when exercise was initiated in the acute phase, continued for 30 days of training, followed by cessation of the exercise training for 30 days. The initial gains were not maintained for the SR following cessation of training for 30 days when initiated in the acute phase of injury (Figure 7.3). The retention of reflex modulation has not been examined when exercise is initiated in the chronic phase of injury. However, the H-reflex gains observed in a chronic patient with a SCI only maintained these gains over a 2-week period after cessation of passive exercise training [7].

INTERVENTIONS: PHARMACOLOGY (L-DOPA, MODAFINIL)

Pharmacologic agents that have been used for patients with SCI have some limitations in treating hyperreflexia in addition to negative side effects. L-Dopa given in a single dose has been investigated in patients following a stroke [27] and in a separate study investigated in patients following SCI [28]. The use of L-Dopa has been reported in normalizing FDD when initiated prior to the onset of hyperreflexia [29]. L-Dopa has also been used in the chronic model of SCI (given once hyperreflexia has been established). This publication [14] reported the H-reflex FDD was normalized following MBET for 60 days, L-Dopa for 60 days, and in a combined group of L-Dopa and MBET [29]. This work confirmed the initial publication that additional exercise was required for an animal with a chronic SCI to show reflex changes. Additional research is needed to investigate the use of L-Dopa in patients with SCI in both the acute and chronic phases of injury.

On the basis of reports in the literature of Modafinil's (MOD) effect on decreasing spasticity in patients with cerebral palsy [30], we sought to quantify the potential therapeutic effects on spasticity in animals following SCI using our previously described reflex measures and to further explore the possible spinal mechanism of action of this antinarcoleptic agent. Additional discussion of the uses of MOD can be found in Chapter 5. In addition to the reduction of spasticity, Hurst [30] also reported that 49% of the children showed improved gait while on MOD.

We investigated the use of daily oral MOD given for 30 days to modulate changes in the H-reflex FDD that have been observed following complete SCI. The animals taking oral MOD (no exercise) as well as the group performing passive exercise, demonstrated changes in the FDD of the H-reflex that were significantly different than transected animals without intervention [18].

Similar to the salutary effects of passive exercise on the H-reflex FDD, daily administration of MOD was shown to prevent the onset of SR windup at 42-days posttransection when compared to transection only animals (Figure 7.3). Like the H-reflex, the normalizing effect of MOD on the SR was compared to the passive exercise group and no statistical difference was found between these two interventions [31]. On the basis of these findings, we filed a patent for the use of MOD for the treatment of hyperreflexia and spasticity and hope to institute clinical trials in the near future.

Having determined the potential therapeutic effect of MOD on spasticity and hyperreflexia, we sought to explore the mechanism behind this action. Another lab within the CTN that focuses on arousal mechanisms had previously determined that MOD increased electrical coupling between reticular activating system cells through the increase in gap junctions (see Chapter 6). Connexin-36 is the primary gap junction in neurons and it has been studied extensively in the brain. Its presence in spinal MN has been found in postnatal mice but declines rapidly [32]. However, electrical coupling has been shown in interneurons of the ventromedial gray matter of the spinal cord that are involved in locomotor control [33].

We examined whole cord as well as regional punches from the lumbar enlargement in animals from various treatment groups and details of these procedures can be found elsewhere [34]. RT-PCR was performed to look for evidence of changes in Cx-36 protein expression across the various interventions. We found evidence that suggests different mechanisms of action for MOD and passive exercise. While both interventions had similar effects on the outcome measures (HR and SR), only MOD-treated animals showed a restoration of Cx-36 levels toward control levels following transection [34]. This finding raises the question of whether combined therapies might have an additive effect in reducing spasticity and hyperreflexia.

CONCLUSIONS

We have utilized outcome measures to quantify hyperreflexia as measured by FDD in both the awake animal and human longitudinally and in terminal experiments in the animal model. Additional outcome measures to quantify spasticity have been utilized and this chapter discussed the literature on the human stretch reflex outcome measure as well as the development of the windup protocol that has been collected on the animal model of complete SCI. A discussion of the difference in the time course for the onset of hyperreflexia and spasticity in the animal model has been identified and suggests different mechanisms that contribute to these symptoms resulting from SCI. We have developed therapeutic avenues and investigated training regimens and use of passive exercise and pharmacologic agents (L-Dopa and Modafinil) in both the acute and chronic phase of SCI. Additional work needs to be done to explore the multiple mechanisms contributing to the symptoms observed following SCI as well as effects of the pharmacologic interventions in the human patient following SCI.

REFERENCES

1. Garcia-Rill E. (1986) The basal ganglia and the locomotor regions. Brain Res 396, 47–63.
2. Iwahara T, Atsuta Y, Garcia-Rill E, Skinner RD. (1991) Locomotion induced by spinal cord stimulation in the neonate rat in vitro. Somatosens Mot Res 8, 281–287.

3. Iwahara T, Atsuta Y, Garcia-Rill E, Skinner RD. (1992) Spinal cord stimulation induced locomotion in the adult cat. Brain Res Bull 28, 99–105.

4. Garcia-Rill E, Skinner RD, Atsuta Y. Method and device for inducing locomotion by electrical stimulation of the spinal cord. Patent number 5,002,053, March 26, 1991.

5. Herman R, He J, D'Luzansky S, Willis W, Dilli S. (2002) Spinal cord stimulation facilitates functional walking in a chronic, incomplete spinal cord injured. Spinal Cord 40, 65–68.

6. Houle JD, Morris K, Skinner RD, Garcia-Rill E, Peterson CA. (1999) Effects of fetal spinal cord tissue transplants and cycling exercise on the soleus muscle in spinalized rats. Muscle Nerve 22, 846–856.

7. Kiser TS, Reese NB, Maresh T, Hearn S, Yates C, Skinner RD, Pait TG, Garcia-Rill E. (2005) Use of a motorized bicycle exercise trainer to normalize frequency-dependent habituation of the H-reflex in spinal cord injury. J Spinal Cord Med 28, 241–245.

8. Reese NB, Skinner RD, Mitchell D, Yates C, Barnes CN, Kiser TS, Garcia-Rill E. (2006) Restoration of frequency-dependent depression of the H-reflex by passive exercise in spinal rats. Spinal Cord 44, 28–34.

9. Malmsten J. (1983) Time course of segmental reflex changes after chronic spinal cord hemisection in the rat. Acta Physiol Scand 119, 435–443.

10. Schindler-Ivens S, Shields RK. (2000) Low frequency depression of H-reflexes in humans with acute and chronic spinal-cord injury. Exp Brain Res 133, 233–241.

11. Curtis DR, Eccles JC. (1960) Synaptic action during and after repetitive stimulation. J Physiol 150, 374–398.

12. Ishikawa K, Ott K, Porter RW, Stuart D. (1966) Low frequency depression of the H wave in normal and spinal man. Exp Neurol 15, 140–156.

13. Skinner RD, Houle JD, Reese NB, Berry CL, Garcia-Rill E. (1996) Effects of exercise and fetal spinal cord implants on the H-reflex in chronically spinalized adult rats. Brain Res 729, 127–131.

14. Arfaj A, Skinner RD, Yates C, Garrison K, Reese ND, Garcia-Rill E. (2009) Reversal of H-reflex hyperactivity by L-dopa and exercise in alert, chronically spinalized rats. Neurosci Abstr 34, 542.11.

15. Thompson FJ, Reier PJ, Lucas CC, Parmer R. (1992) Altered patterns of reflex excitability subsequent to contusion injury of the rat spinal cord. J Neurophysiol 68, 1473–1486.

16. Yates CC, Charlesworth A, Reese NB, Skinner RD, Garcia-Rill E. (2008) The effects of passive exercise therapy initiated prior to or after the development of hyperreflexia following spinal transection. Exp Neurol 213, 405–409.

17. Nielsen JB, Crone C, Hultborn H. (2007) The spinal pathophysiology of spasticity–from a basic science point of view. Acta Physiol (Oxf) 189, 171–180.

18. Yates CC, Charlesworth A, Reese NB, Ishida K, Skinner RD, Garcia-Rill E. (2009) Modafinil normalized hyperreflexia after spinal transection in adult rats. Spinal Cord 47, 481–485.

19. Voerman GE, Gregoric M, Hermens HJ. (2005) Neurophysiological methods for the assessment of spasticity: the Hoffmann reflex, the tendon reflex, and the stretch reflex. Disabil Rehabil 27, 33–68.

20. Johnson GR. (2002) Outcome measures of spasticity. Eur J Neurol 9(suppl 1), 10–16; Discussion 53–61.
21. Hornby TG, Kahn JH, Wu M, Schmit BD. (2006) Temporal facilitation of spastic stretch reflexes following human spinal cord injury. J Physiol 571, 593–604.
22. Bennett DJ, Sanelli L, Cooke CL, Harvey PJ, Gorassini MA. (2004) Spastic Long-Lasting Reflexes in the Awake Rat After Sacral Spinal Cord Injury. J Neurophysiol 91, 2247–2258.
23. Murray KC, Nakae A, Stephens MJ, Rank M, D'Amico J, Harvey PJ, Li X, Harris RL, Ballou EW, Anelli R, Heckman CJ, Mashimo T, Vavrek R, Sanelli L, Gorassini MA, Bennett DJ, Fouad K. (2010) Recovery of motoneuron and locomotor function after spinal cord injury depends on constitutive activity in 5-HT2C receptors. Nat Med 16, 694–700.
24. Yates C, Garrison K, Reese NB, Charlesworth A, Garcia-Rill E. (2011) Novel mechanism for hyperreflexia and spasticity. Prog Brain Res 188, 167–180.
25. Norrie BA, Nevett-Duchcherer JM, Gorassini MA. (2005) Reduced functional recovery by delaying motor training after spinal cord injury. J Neurophysiol 94, 255–264.
26. Phadke CP, Flynn SM, Thompson FJ, Behrman AL, Trimble MH, Kukulka CG. (2009) Comparison of single bout effects of bicycle training versus locomotor training on paired reflex depression of the soleus H-reflex after motor incomplete spinal cord injury. Arch Phys Med Rehabil 90, 1218–1228.
27. Crisostomo EA, Duncan PW, Propst M, Dawson DV, Davis JN. (1988) Evidence that amphetamine with physical therapy promotes recovery of motor function in stroke patients. Ann Neurol 23, 94–97.
28. Eriksson J, Olausson B, Jankowska E. (1996) Antispastic effects of L-dopa. Exp Brain Res 111, 296–304.
29. Liu H, Skinner RD, Arfaj A, Yates C, Reese NB, Williams K, Garcia-Rill E. (2010) l-Dopa effect on frequency-dependent depression of the H-reflex in adult rats with complete spinal cord transection. Brain Res Bull 83, 262–265.
30. Hurst DL, Lajara-Nanson WA, Lance-Fish ME. (2006) Walking with modafinil and its use in diplegic cerebral palsy: retrospective review. J Child Neurol 21, 294–297.
31. Garrison MK, Yates CC, Reese NB, Skinner RD, Garcia-Rill E. (2011) Wind-up of stretch reflexes as a measure of spasticity in chronic spinalized rats: The effects of passive exercise and modafinil. Exp Neurol 227, 104–109.
32. Walton KD, Navarrete R. (1991) Postnatal changes in motoneurone electrotonic coupling studied in the in vitro rat lumbar spinal cord. J Physiol 433, 283–305.
33. Hinckley CA, Ziskind-Conhaim L. (2006) Electrical coupling between locomotor-related excitatory interneurons in the mammalian spinal cord. J Neurosci 26, 8477–8483.
34. Yates C, Garrison MK, Reese NB, Garcia-Rill E. (2010) Therapeutic approaches for spinal cord Injury induced spasticity. Translational Neurosci 1, 160–169.

8 Translational Research in Neonatology

Richard Whit Hall

INTRODUCTION

Translational research has played a key role in the care of our most vulnerable population—neonates. This chapter will explore the translation of animal research to the prevention and cure of human disease. The benefit and harm of delaying promising research findings in animal models to human care will also be explored, along with barriers that will need to be addressed if we are to make use of the rapid explosion of biomedical research. The chapter will then assess the translation of research findings in academic health centers to the community hospital, so-called T2 research. Most neonatal care takes place in community hospitals, far away from academia. Thus, better practices in training institutions must translate into better care for everyone if the population as a whole is going to experience improved outcomes. Additionally, the experience and knowledge of practicing clinicians must be taken into account to generate useful research. Finally, solutions for these perplexing problems will be explored.

Neonatology has experienced the thrill of victory and the agony of defeat. There have been huge improvements in outcomes interspersed with catastrophic setbacks. For example, in the 1950s, the widespread use of oxygen led to an epidemic of retinopathy of prematurity, followed by an epidemic of cerebral palsy when its use was too severely restricted [1]. The widespread use of chloramphenicol led to the "gray baby syndrome" because no pharmacokinetic studies had been done in the neonatal population [2] and neurological dysfunction resulted from the routine use of hexachlorophene in newborns [3]. On the other hand, neonatology has sometimes delayed translating promising findings in animal research to human infants and from human studies to the general population. For example, in 1969, Liggins found that betamethasone, when infused prior

Translational Neuroscience: A Guide to a Successful Program, First Edition. Edited by Edgar Garcia-Rill.
© 2012 John Wiley & Sons, Inc. Published 2012 by John Wiley & Sons, Inc.

to the delivery of preterm lambs, would ameliorate the symptoms of hyaline membrane disease in preterm animals [4]. He followed this work in humans in 1972, finding that betamethasone, when given to mothers in preterm labor, resulted in less hyaline membrane disease and improved survival in preterm neonates [5]. In 1994, after thousands of neonatal deaths and intracranial hemorrhages in survivors, the NIH released a Consensus Development Conference Statement, supported by the American College of Obstetrics and Gynecology, that stated that mothers with threatened preterm delivery should receive *antenatal* steroids. While antenatal steroids were adopted soon after that, there has been concern among the neonatology community regarding the delay in the use of this powerful ally in the fight against the complications of prematurity.

In 2001, after the use of *postnatal* steroids for chronic lung disease had become widespread, a meta-analysis found that the only benefit from these drugs was a transient benefit in pulmonary mechanics [6]. Unfortunately, they were also found to be associated with dramatic increases in neurodevelopmental impairment, and their use was almost entirely abandoned [6]. These two scenarios, one a delay in translating promising research into clinical adaptation and the other the adoption of unproven therapies too quickly, demonstrate the difficulties in translating research into human benefit. Good translational research is difficult.

THE NEED FOR NEONATAL RESEARCH

Despite a call for more research in the neonatal population, especially in pharmacotherapy, there has not been as much investment as was planned. Currently, only 10% of all drugs used in neonates have Food and Drug Administration (FDA) approval. Further, because human development changes so much between the time of viability (23 weeks postmenstrual age) and term (40 weeks postmenstrual age), research that may be applicable to a younger group of neonates may not be applicable to an older group of infants. The rigors of practicing neonatology, because of the emphasis on clinical care, leave little time for research interests. This puts the practicing neonatal clinician scientist at a disadvantage. How can we improve?

THE BUILDING BLOCKS: BASIC RESEARCH

Socrates believed that science was the foundation of philosophy. Translational research, like philosophy, is built upon good basic science. It allows scientists to develop plausible hypotheses, mechanisms of action, and possible new therapies. This is well illustrated by the Human Genome Project, which mapped the 46 human chromosomes and led to the development of targeted gene therapies, targeted cancer risks, prenatal diagnosis of serious or lethal conditions, and the whole realm of genomics in drug therapy [7]. On the other hand, some diseases, such as schizophrenia, still need good basic science research to elucidate the cause(s) of this devastating disease. While it is known that prenatal nutrition and infection are important in brain development, how those may affect the propensity to schizophrenia and other psychiatric illnesses is unknown [8]. Thus, there is a real need to study the basic science of mental illness.

Animal studies have elucidated the basic mechanisms of many neonatal diseases, but animal models pose obstacles in research. For example, a rat pup weighs only 5–7 g at birth. Although, at birth, rat pups are considered to be consistent gestationally with a 23-week human fetus, they are clearly more mature than the human at birth in many areas such as bowel maturity and brain development. Finding the appropriate animal model with coinciding developmental stages to the fragile neonate is difficult. The human central nervous system at birth, for example, is complex compared with animal species. Yet, we study these models to help elucidate mechanisms of central nervous system development in rat models, making inferences that are (supposedly) applicable to human development. Developing appropriate models in neonatology is difficult and clearly challenging to basic science investigators.

PUPS TO BABIES AND BACK AGAIN: T1 RESEARCH

Despite the problems noted in the preceding text, animal studies yield critical information that can be taken from the laboratory to the bedside. Rat pups have been shown to reveal some of the mechanisms behind adverse neurodevelopmental outcome in chronic pain states and the effects of treatment on those outcomes [9]. Another animal model, the preterm rabbit, was critical in the development of treatments for the lung diseases commonly affecting neonates. This model has been useful in assessing therapies for hyaline membrane disease, meconium aspiration syndrome, mechanical ventilation, and other diseases affecting the human newborn pulmonary system. The model was critical in the discovery of surfactant and its surfactant-associated proteins, which was later trialed in preterm human neonates [10,11]. This discovery was arguably the most dramatic finding of the last two decades for neonatology. Other animal models have included the baboon for bronchopulmonary dysplasia, which illuminated much of the pathophysiology for the most expensive disease affecting preterm neonates [12], and the neonatal swine model, which has been useful in evaluating neonatal skin [13], and cardiac dysfunction. Thus, animal studies are critical to the advancement of neonatology. What are the keys to translating the knowledge gained in animal models to neonatal care?

NO PROBLEM CAN BE SOLVED UNLESS IT IS FIRST IDENTIFIED

Practicing clinicians must articulate the clinical problems facing neonatal specialists, and they must be able to assimilate the data from basic science research. The only way progress will be made is to facilitate the free flow of ideas across disciplines. Frequent informal meetings must be a priority for translational T1 research to be successful. The unique clinical difficulties facing neonatologists provide exciting research opportunities, but they must be identified. After a problem is identified, a methodical approach involving clinical and basic science disciplines should be discussed. There will never be enough resources to solve every problem facing neonatal practitioners, but the problems can be prioritized to areas that are important and are known strengths of the institution. Then, the approach can be discussed, and the decision of whether or not to invest in solving a clinical problem can be evaluated in a systematic manner (see Table 8.1). Following the step-by-step process outlined in the table will pave the way for a more effective plan of research when using animal models.

The specific concerns surrounding neonatal translational research include the following:

1. Despite a push for more research in this population, there is apprehension about doing research on vulnerable populations, especially neonates, among health care providers and parents. Taking the results of animal studies and applying those results to human neonates is challenging.
2. Institutional Review Boards remain cautious regarding newborn research, especially when the translation goes from animal work to humans.
3. The FDA requires preliminary data in neonates, even if these have already been obtained in infants or children. If approval from the FDA

Table 8.1   Steps involved in a successful translational research project in neonatology

Step 1	Identify a problem related to newborn care.
Step 2	Discuss with relevant faculty (must be involved in pediatric research).
Step 3	Prioritize idea: is the problem important to neonatology? Is the evaluation an institutional strength?
Step 4	Discuss pros and cons with basic and clinical researchers. Is there a neonatal animal model?
Step 5	Discuss method for evaluation.
Step 6	Discuss funding. NICHD is highly competitive. Is there another source?
Step 7	Discuss what can be expected from the research.
Step 8	Discuss the trials in the neonatal population. *Is this safe in neonates?* Will there be problems getting Review Board approval? Will this require approval from the FDA?

must be obtained, the process can be delayed for 2–3 years, costing thousands of dollars. The FDA is a regulatory agency that is charged with numerous duties, now including protection of the food supply. Thus, the agency is more familiar with drug companies and commercial enterprises than academic researchers. The FDA will be very cautious when approving translational research in humans. Thus, preliminary data are often obtained from the clinical application of therapies in neonates (in which case there are no controlled experiments involving animals and/or humans). In summary, translation of animal research to human neonates is more difficult because animal models are often small, they must be appropriate for the gestational age being studied, and human neonates are a vulnerable population. Despite these difficulties, building translational research on good basic science, developing good communication between animal researchers and clinical practitioners, and careful selection of the animal model will result in excellence in translational research.

FROM THE BEDSIDE TO THE COMMUNITY: T2 RESEARCH

Just as basic science discoveries in the laboratory using animal models are critical to the success of translational research in neonatology, so is disseminating evidence-based practices from the patient bedside to the community at large. In this way, patterns and practices of care can be changed to improve the health of all.

One of the greatest failures of neonatology is the inability or unwillingness to translate the life-saving benefits of regionalization of neonatal intensive care into practice. The failure to regionalize care and deliver high-risk pregnancies in perinatal centers is associated with increased morbidity and mortality [14–16]. Thus, rates of neonatal survival have improved in some countries (e.g., Canada) but not in the United States, despite significant improvements in technology [17]. A regionalized perinatal care system can dramatically improve the outcomes of very low birth weight (VLBW) neonates. For example, neonatal outcomes are directly related to the level of care and census of the neonatal intensive care units (NICUs) in which they are treated [15,16,18]. In Arkansas, if the goals of Toward Improving the Outcome of Pregnancy (TIOP) III were achieved, more than 80% of all VLBW neonates would deliver in level 3 units, decreasing infant mortality by 0.8/1000 [19] (see Figure 8.1). Unfortunately, many states, including Arkansas, either do not use these designated nursery levels in their system of perinatal care or they do not abide by these designations [20,21], despite a publication history of over 30 years [22]. A recent analysis of 19 states found that the number of VLBW neonates delivering at level 3 centers varied from 64% to 93% [21]. The goal of delivering an adequate number of VLBW neonates in level 3 centers has been achieved by only

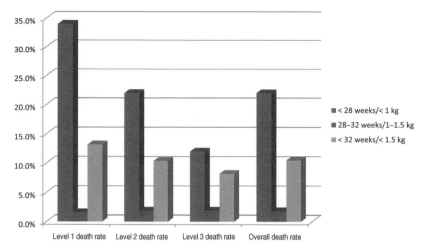

Figure 8.1   Mortality rate. Note the increased mortality rate in neonates <1 kg in the lower level nurseries compared with the level 3 nursery. *$p < 0.001$ for babies < 1000 g and/or < 28 weeks in level 3 nurseries compared with level 1 or 2 nurseries. (For color detail, please see the color plate section.)

five states [23]. If Phibbs et al. are correct, delivering more VLBW neonates in larger centers could save thousands of lives annually [18]. Unfortunately, the solution is not as simple as recommending or requiring that all preterm pregnancies deliver at centers with larger NICUs. In the real world, many pregnant women present to smaller hospitals with conditions that require emergent/urgent delivery, that is, prolapsed cord, placental abruption, and advanced labor, which precludes safe transfer to a larger center. With these deliveries, there is inadequate time to receive prenatal steroids, which also leads to increased mortality and morbidity [24]. Numerous factors such as inadequate prenatal care [25], parental and cultural preferences [26,27], financial considerations and distance [28] to the referral center are associated with nonreferral. Additionally, there are subtle "town-gown" rivalries that discourage transfer to academic medical centers from community hospitals (although these rivalries can be overcome) [29]. Finally, local hospitals enjoy widespread support from their communities, as most parents believe that it is "very important" to deliver close to their support systems [30]. Countries such as Australia, where there is less pressure to deregionalize [31], are able to successfully transfer up to 90% of their high-risk mothers to the appropriate hospital, even though transport distances are large (sometimes over 500 miles). The United States has not been as successful. It is unknown whether this is because of factors that are generally uncontrollable, due to greater distances between community and regional centers, due to pressures in the United States to deregionalize, or due to poor communication between smaller and larger hospitals.

Because of these barriers, many patients who might otherwise be referred to a center with a higher level of care are kept in smaller hospitals. Because regionalization of care implies transfer of patients away from their primary care providers, and often their families and social support, patients and providers are reluctant to transfer [32,33]. The obvious findings of regionalization of neonatal intensive care must be translated into practice.

Taking the findings from the academic bedside to the community where most of neonatology is practiced can be challenging, but just as important is taking the findings from the community to academia. Community health care providers provide tremendous insight, patient material, and judgment to the health care system. It is imperative that these providers become involved in the process of translating research into clinical care. A dictatorial stance that only goes from the ivory tower of academia to community providers will not be successful, and it will, understandably, alienate and eliminate cooperation with community physicians. Telemedicine has been used successfully to engage practicing community neonatologists. The program includes weekly pediatric telemedicine educational conferences and tri-weekly census rounds (see Chapter 9) from the nursery that are truly interactive, with consultation going in both directions. One of the most successful educational conferences was presented by one of the community providers from his patient population. He successfully brought in pediatric residents, subspecialists, and practicing general pediatricians, a collaborative effort.

This type of interaction can influence care. The spell out TOUCH initiative, which was a telemedicine program connecting nine hospital labor and delivery suites and nurseries with the one large perinatal institution, made an impact on regionalization of neonatal care. In the TOUCH initiative, delivery patterns shifted so that fewer high-risk pregnancies delivered in hospitals that were not equipped to care for their babies (see Table 8.2).

Table 8.2   Delivery patterns during TOUCH

	Telemedicine hospital—no NICU number (%)	Telemedicine hospital—with NICU number (%)	Nontelemedicine hospital—no NICU number (%)	Nontelemedicine hospital—with NICU number (%)
Pretelemedicine	**50 (13.05)**	25 (6.53)	90 (23.50)	102 (26.63)
Posttelemedicine	**27 (7.03)***	33 (8.69)	91 (23.70)	111 (28.91)

Note: "NICU" hospitals were defined as having a neonatologist and could provide assisted ventilation; "no NICU" hospitals did not have neonatology coverage and could not provide prolonged assisted ventilation.
*$p = 0.075$ chi square for change in distribution of delivery hospitals between the before and after telemedicine intervention.
NICU, neonatal intensive care unit.

Table 8.3   **NICU hospitals were defined as in the preceding text**

Delivery hospital		Deceased number (%)	Home number (%)	Transferred number (%)
TM hospital—no NICU	Pre $n = 46$	6 (13)	19 (32.61)	21 (46)
	Post $n = 27$	2 (6.7)*	9 (33.33)	16 (59)
TM hospital—with NICU	Pre $n = 24$	1 (4.2)	20 (80)	3 (13)
	Post $n = 33$	3 (9.1)	26 (79)	4 (12)
Non-TM hospital—no NICU	Pre $n = 86$	11 (13)	17 (20)	58 (67)
	Post $n = 87$	6 (6.9)	16 (18)	65 (75)
Non-TM hospital—with NICU	Pre $n = 102$	13 (13)	74 (73)	15 (15)
	Post $n = 108$	7 (6.5)	84 (78)	17 (16)

Note: "Pre" represents the period before and "post" represents the period after beginning telemedicine. Note the decreases in mortality in the telemedicine equipped non-NICU hospitals.
*$p = 0.106$ t-test before and after comparison within hospital group.

This type of translational research can save lives (see Table 8.3). We can safely say that the Telemedicine Core Facility (described in Chapter 9) we established, has solved the problem of regionalization for the entire state, has decreased the mortality rate in VLBW babies, and has decreased the incidence of intraventricular hemorrhage that costs the state at least $1.5 million per year.

THE ROLE OF COMPARATIVE EFFECTIVENESS RESEARCH

Another valuable method of taking the findings from the bedside to the community is through comparative effectiveness research (CER). CER has been defined as "the conduct and synthesis of research comparing the benefits and harms of different interventions and strategies to prevent, diagnose, treat, and monitor health conditions in 'real world' settings." This methodology holds promise for research in pregnancy and preterm birth, priority conditions identified by the Medicare Prescription Drug, Improvement, and Modernization Act, because of the diverse populations involved and the need to study their care in real-world settings, that is, not just in academic centers [34,35]. Neonatology has three research networks: the NICHD Network (a consortium of 16 academic NICUs), the Vermont-Oxford Network (>800 academic, community, and private NICUs around the world), and Pediatrix (>250 private NICUs). Obstetrics has the NICHD Maternal-Fetal Medicine Units Network, consisting of 14 academic obstetrical units. A limitation of all the networks, however, is that they are not population based. Their focus is, appropriately, the care of neonates in their nurseries. Research must focus on a defined population to make the translation of findings relevant to the "real world." The principles of CER include cost-effectiveness, relevant population-based studies, and statistical methodology such as high-dimensional propensity scoring and instrumental variable analysis, which should be applied in populations, not just in certain centers [36].

Three such examples of how the principles of CER have been applied to entire populations are described later and illustrate the impact that such a wide-reaching focus can have on neonatal patients. One example of CER is a neonatal program called the *Newborn Screening Translational Research Network*. This research network seeks to stimulate research in medical genetics [37]. Congenital defects account for approximately one-third of all infant deaths, and great strides have been made in identifying inborn errors of metabolism through newborn screening using tandem mass spectrometry. Just a few years ago, phenylketonuria was the only metabolic disorder screened for in the nursery. Now, most states screen for 29 or more disorders as recommended by the American College of Genetics. However, individually, these disorders are rare, but taken together, they account for a significant portion of neonatal deaths. The results of enhanced newborn screening have been astounding, but many questions remain that can only be addressed with a large population base. Some of the unanswered questions include knowledge about the natural history of some of the disorders, how to prevent or treat other disorders, identification of benign (or severe) variants of common disorders, and the effect of positive screening with negative confirmatory tests on parental anxiety and attachment. Only a large translational research network as described in the preceding text with an adequate patient base can address these problems.

Another example that encompasses an international translational research focus is EuroPrevail that is a multi-institutional birth cohort study. Since the true incidence of food allergies in children is unknown, it will address the prevalence of food allergies by utilizing the diagnostic gold standard, a double blind placebo-controlled food challenge test. This initiative will provide data on prevalence, risk factors, quality of life, and costs of food allergies in Europe, which will lead to the development of better treatment strategies for children. Only through such a large birth cohort with representation from different regions of Europe, will the true prevalence of food allergies be known. Clearly, the results of this study will be applicable to the children of the United States as well [38].

The third example involves The Johns Hopkins Research Institute who partnered with Phil Thuma from the Macha Mission in Zambia, Africa. Dr. Thuma set a goal of eradicating malaria within 8 years. In 2003, there were 80–100 infant deaths per year in the Macha Mission area, along with several more cases of cerebral malaria resulting in permanent brain damage and over 1000 admissions per year of children with anemia due to malaria. In 2009, in the Macha Mission Hospital, there were only 40 admissions of children with malaria and only 2 deaths. Translational research brought about this dramatic change. Before translation of the research findings into clinical practice, the epidemiology of the disease and its prevalence had to be understood. Then, the mosquito vector for this disease, the Anopheles Mosquito, and its habits had to be understood. The treatment, chloroquine, had to be developed and finally, there had to be understanding of the culture of the people in and around the Macha Mission [39]. Only after the background research was accomplished, could the findings be translated into clinical care. This project illustrates several points regarding translational research. First, it is rewarding. To save that many lives over 8 years is an incredible benefit to the people of Africa. Second, the basic research had to be done before the findings could be translated into clinical practice. Next, the project took time, 8 years, before there was any benefit. And finally, the translation of the research findings into clinical practice had to be done in a culturally sensitive manner. It will require an even greater effort to translate the findings from this community to Zambia, the home country of the Macha Mission, and the other nations of Africa.

The aforementioned examples illustrate why CER must be based on sound science; it must be population based; it takes time; and it can be extremely rewarding. Thus, CER is an effective means of doing translational research.

BARRIERS AND REWARDS IN TRANSLATIONAL RESEARCH IN NEONATOLOGY

Neonatology is a demanding clinical specialty. NICU patients demand a great deal of time, which takes away from the time that could be devoted to research. Further, the reimbursement for clinical care in neonatal medicine is high compared with many other specialties, and (in the author's opinion) the rewards are great in clinical care as well. Thus, the lure of clinical work in neonatology is attractive in both private practice and in academic medicine. In order to participate in translational research, clinician scientists *must* have the insight that can only come from involvement in neonatal care [40]. Because of time constraints and other barriers, there are inadequate numbers of neonatologists who are willing to be clinician scientists and forego some of the clinical rewards.

Despite these barriers, there are great opportunities to participate in translational research in neonatology. Neonatal training programs now emphasize research over clinical care. In a 3-year neonatal fellowship, there are 22 months devoted to research and 14 months devoted to clinical neonatology. Thus, training programs emphasize research as a prerequisite to becoming a neonatologist. Additionally, the patient population in neonatology tends to be more uniform than in other specialties. Additionally, since much of neonatology is related to preterm birth, a common neonatal condition, findings in this population can be translated to many other neonatal patients.

OPPORTUNITIES FOR TRANSLATIONAL RESEARCH IN NEONATOLOGY

There are many opportunities to translate findings in this population to the community, such as regionalization of perinatal care. Another example is the use of folic acid to prevent neural tube defects. In order to prevent birth defects, folic acid must be taken close to or before the time of conception, usually before the mother knows she is pregnant. Thus, most mothers (approximately 2/3) do not take the vitamin in time to prevent spina bifida and other neural tube defects. However, food fortification has been effective in providing adequate vitamin supplementation to prevent one of the most dreaded congenital anomalies affecting neonates, especially in poor and undereducated mothers [41,42]. Translating these findings into improved patient outcomes is an outstanding opportunity to prove the worth of translational research in neonatology. Another reason for opportunity in neonatal translational research is the patient population. These babies are usually hospitalized in larger centers with academic leanings. Thus, they are easier to access and they contribute a large number of potential research subjects. In summary, while there are challenges in attracting and keeping talented clinician scientists, there are wonderful opportunities and rewards for participating in translational research in neonatology that can save countless lives.

CONCLUSION

Translational research is critical if neonatology is to continue to advance. Good translational research is built upon good basic science, and taking the findings from animal models to human infants is a necessary step to improve care. There are significant barriers to translational research in neonatology, including developing appropriate animal models, matching those models for gestational age and (since neonates are a vulnerable population) translating findings in animals to human infants. On the other hand, there is ample opportunity to improve neonatal clinical care through translational research. Neonatology training emphasizes research and the neonatal population has a high volume of patients, many of whom are located in academic institutions. And there are outstanding opportunities to take the findings from the bedside to the community to improve infant mortality and decrease congenital defects. Translational research will continue to move neonatology forward.

REFERENCES

1. Silverman WA. (1968) Oxygen therapy and retrolental fibroplasia. Amer J Public Health Nations Health. 58, 2009–2011.
2. Feder HM, Jr., Osier C, Maderazo EG. (1981) Chloramphenicol: a review of its use in clinical practice. Rev Infect Dis 3, 479–491.
3. Anderson JM, Cockburn F, Forfar JO, Harkness RA, Kelly RW, Kilshaw B. (1981) Neonatal spongiform myelinopathy after restricted application of hexachlorophane skin disinfectant. J Clin Pathol 34, 25–29.
4. Liggins GC. Premature delivery of foetal lambs infused with glucocorticoids. (1969) J Endocrinol 45, 515–523.
5. Liggins GC, Howie RN. (1972) A controlled trial of antepartum glucocorticoid treatment for prevention of the respiratory distress syndrome in premature infants. Pediatrics 50, 515–525.
6. Barrington KJ. (2001) The adverse neuro-developmental effects of postnatal steroids in the preterm infant: a systematic review of RCTs. BMC Pediatrics 1, 1–9.
7. McBride CM, Guttmacher AE. (2009) Commentary: trailblazing a research agenda at the interface of pediatrics and genomic discovery–a commentary on the psychological aspects of genomics and child health. J Pediat Psychol 34, 662–664.
8. McGrath JJ, Richards LJ. (2009) Why schizophrenia epidemiology needs neurobiology–and vice versa. Schizophr Bull 35, 577–581.
9. Rovnaghi CR, Garg S, Hall RW, Bhutta BT, Anand KJ. (2008) Ketamine analgesia for inflammatory pain in neonatal rats: a factorial randomized trial examining long-term effect. Behav Brain Funct 4, 35–44.
10. Ohama Y, Ogawa Y. (1999) Treatment of meconium aspiration syndrome with surfactant lavage in an experimental rabbit model. Pediat Pulmonol 28, 18–23.
11. Ohashi T, Polk D, Ikegami M, Ueda T, Jobe A. (1994) Ontogeny and effects of exogenous surfactant treatment on SP-A, SP-B, and SP-C mRNA expression in rabbit lungs. Amer J Physiol 267, L46–L51.
12. Morton RL, Das KC, Guo XL, Ikle DN, White CW. (1999) Effect of oxygen on lung superoxide dismutase activities in premature baboons with bronchopulmonary dysplasia. Amer J Physiol 276, L64–L74.
13. Zhang Z, Monteiro-Riviere NA. (1997) Comparison of integrins in human skin, pig skin, and perfused skin: an in vitro skin toxicology model. J Appl Toxicol 17, 247–253.
14. Mauch J, Kutter APN, Madjdpour C, Spielmann N, Balmer C, Frotzler A, Bettschart-Wolfensberger R, Weiss M. (2010) Electrocardiographic changes during continuous intravenous application of bupivacaine in neonatal pigs. Brit J Anaesth 105, 437–441.
15. Lasswell SM, Barfield WD, Rochat RW, Blackmon L. (2010) Perinatal regionalization for very low-birth-weight and very preterm infants: a meta-analysis. JAMA 304, 992–1000.
16. Palmer KG, Kronsberg SS, Barton BA, Hobbs CA, Hall RW, Anand KJ. (2005) Effect of inborn versus outborn delivery on clinical outcomes in ventilated preterm neonates: secondary results from the NEOPAIN trial. J Perinatol 25, 270–275.

17. Joseph KS, Liston RM, Dodds L, Dahlgren L, Allen AC. (2007) Socioeconomic status and perinatal outcomes in a setting with universal access to essential health care services. Can Med Assoc J 177, 583–590.

18. Phibbs CS, Baker LC, Caughey AB, Danielsen B, Schmitt SK, Phibbs RH. (2007) Level and volume of neonatal intensive care and mortality in very-low-birth-weight infants. New Eng J Med 356, 2165–2175.

19. Nugent R, Golden WE, Hall R, Bronstein J, Grimes D, Lowery C. (2011) Locations and outcomes of premature births in Arkansas. J Ark Med Soc 107, 258–259.

20. Blackmon L, Barfield W, Stark A. (2009) Hospital neonatal services in the United States: variation in definitions, criteria, and regulatory status, 2008. J Perinatol 29, 788–794.

21. Neonatal intensive-care unit admission of infants with very low birth weight—19 States. (2006). Morb Mortal Wkly Rep (2010) 59, 1444–1447.

22. National Committee on Perinatal Health. (1976) Toward Improving the Outcome of Pregnancy. White Plains, NY: National Foundation-March of Dimes.

23. Maternal and Child Health Bureau: Multi-Year Report, Performance Measure #17 Health Resources and Services Administration, US Department of Health and Human Services. (2009) Accessed February 1, 2010, at https://perfdatahrsagov/mchb/tvisreports/MeasurementData/Standard NationalMeasureIndicatorSearchaspx?MeasureType=Performance&Year Type=MultiYear.

24. Delaney-Black V, Lubchenco LO, Butterfield LJ, Goldson E, Koops BL, Lazotte DC. (1989) Outcome of very-low-birth-weight infants: are populations of neonates inherently different after antenatal versus neonatal referral? Amer J Obstet Gynecol 160, 545–552.

25. Attar MA, Hanrahan K, Lang SW, Gates MR, Bratton SL. (2006) Pregnant mothers out of the perinatal regionalization's reach. J Perinatol 26, 210–214.

26. Bracht M, Kandankery A, Nodwell S, Stade B. (2002) Cultural differences and parental responses to the preterm infant at risk: strategies for supporting families. Neonatal Netw 21, 31–38.

27. Samuelson JL, Buehler JW, Norris D, Sadek R. (2002) Maternal characteristics associated with place of delivery and neonatal mortality rates among very-low-birthweight infants, Georgia. Paediat Perinatal Epidemiol 16, 305–313.

28. Gessner BD, Muth PT. (2001) Perinatal care regionalization and low birth weight infant mortality rates in Alaska. Amer J Obstet Gynecol 185, 623–628.

29. Johnston GM, Murnaghan D, Buehler SK, Nugent LS. (1998) Atlantic Breast Cancer Information Project: formation of a "town-gown" partnership. Cancer Prevent Control 2, 23–29.

30. Martucci M. (2004) Considerations in planning a newborn developmental care program in a community hospital setting. Adv Neonatal Care 4, 59–66.

31. Lui K, Abdel-Latif ME, Allgood CL, Allgood CL, Bajuk B, Oei J, Berry A, Henderson-Smart D, New South, Wales Australian Capital Territory Neonatal Intensive Care Unit Study, Group. (2006) Improved outcomes of extremely premature outborn infants: effects of strategic changes in perinatal and retrieval services. Pediatrics 118, 2076–2083.

32. Hall-Barrow J, Hall RW, Burke BL, Jr. (2009) Telemedicine and neonatal regionalization of care—ensuring that the right baby gets to the right nursery. Pediatric Ann 38, 557–561.

33. Hall R, Bronstein J, Fallon A, Nugent R, McGhee J. (2009) Can telemedicine be used to improve neonatal and infant mortality in a medicaid population in a rural state. Abstract, Pediatric Academic Society. http://www.abstracts2view.com/pasall/view.php?nu=PAS09L1_1879

34. Sox HC, Greenfield S. (2009) Comparative effectiveness research: a report from the Institute of Medicine. Ann Intern Med 151, 203–205.

35. Chalkidou K, Whicher D, Kary W, Tunis S. (2009) Comparative effectiveness research priorities: identifying critical gaps in evidence for clinical and health policy decision making. Int J Technol Assess Health Care 25, 241–248.

36. Schneeweiss S. (2007) Developments in post-marketing comparative effectiveness research. Clin Pharmacol Ther 82, 143–156.

37. Levy HL. Newborn screening conditions: what we know, what we do not know, and how we will know it. Genet Med. 2010; 12: S213–S214.

38. Keil T, McBride D, Grimshaw K, Niggemann B, Xepapadaki P, Zannikos K, Sigurdardottir ST, Clausen M, Reche M, Pascual C, Stanczyk AP, Kowalski ML, Dubakiene R, Drasutiene G, Roberts G, Schoemaker AFA, Sprikkelman AB, Fiocchi A, Martelli A, Dufour S, Hourihane J, Kulig M, Wjst M, Yazdanbakhsh M, Szepfalusi Z, van Ree R, Willich SN, Wahn U, Mills ENC, Beyer K. (2010) The multinational birth cohort of EuroPrevall: background, aims and methods. Allergy 65, 482–490.

39. Thuma PE, van Dijk J, Bucala R, Debebe Z, Nekhai S, Kuddo T, Nouraie M, Weiss G, Gordeuk VR. (2011) Distinct clinical and immunologic profiles in severe malarial anemia and cerebral malaria in Zambia. J Infect Dis 203, 211–219.

40. Ward RM, Lane RH, Albertine KH. (2006) Basic and translational research in neonatal pharmacology. J Perinatol 26(Suppl 2), S8–S12.

41. Knudsen VK, Orozova-Bekkevold I, Rasmussen LB, Mikkelsen TB, Michaelsen KF, Olsen SF. (2004) Low compliance with recommendations on folic acid use in relation to pregnancy: is there a need for fortification? Public Health Nutr 7, 843–850.

42. Finglas PM, de Meer K, Molloy A, Verhoef P, Pietrzik K, Powers HJ, van der Straeten D, Jägerstad M, Varela-Moreiras G, van Vliet T, Havenaar R, Buttriss J, Wright AJ. (2006) Research goals for folate and related B vitamin in Europe. Eur J Clin Nutrition 60, 287–294.

9 Telemedicine in Translational Neuroscience

Amy Ballard and Richard Whit Hall

Community-based research usually entails direct interaction between the clinician scientist and the public. It encompasses the evaluation of research questions in the community setting, such as the evaluation of hypertension in the community; it can involve the evaluation of medical knowledge in a community setting, such as an evaluation of a pamphlet on birth control for adolescents; or community-based research can imply an evaluation of the dissemination of medical care into the community. Telemedicine is an excellent example of the latter. Community-based research is geared toward optimizing medical practice so that the "community" is the actual guiding force behind the way that health care is delivered and how it evolves. Through the interchange between clinician scientists and the public, consensus guidelines for treatment can be developed in order to provide the most successful and cost-effective diagnostic approaches, treatment options, and follow-up procedures. In targeting health care professionals, the implementation of new and more effective therapies can also be enhanced. As a result, the overall health of the population can be effectively improved through community-based research, in which the "community" is health care providers.

Boosting adoption of best practices of health care in the community is a major tenet of translational research. However, several factors must be in place for this to be achieved. First of all, a consensus must be reached on what is considered "best practices." Once that is identified, then determining the most efficient way to implement these practices must occur, and that involves considering best modes of communication in order to ensure that such practices are actually applied to patient care. Finally, effectiveness research needs to be implemented in order to confirm that medical practices are indeed being optimized.

Telemedicine is a powerful tool that shows tremendous promise in facilitating the steps necessary for successful identification and implementation

Translational Neuroscience: A Guide to a Successful Program, First Edition. Edited by Edgar Garcia-Rill.
© 2012 John Wiley & Sons, Inc. Published 2012 by John Wiley & Sons, Inc.

123

of best practices. Telemedicine is the electronic exchange of medical information or data that may consist of high-resolution images, written medical histories and data, or specialty consult through various modes of technological communication between individuals at different locations.

HISTORY OF TELEMEDICINE

Although telemedicine may seem like a new concept, it has been in existence since remote communication devices were invented. For example, the inception of the telegraph in the 1800s was used to communicate medical emergencies and to request medical help. Then, the invention of the telephone in 1876 enabled two-way audible communication that was used as a way to seek medical consultation, advice, and support as well as assisting the patient and patient's family in his or her overall care. In fact, the telephone continues to serve as the predominant mode of transmission of many diagnostic tools such as electrocardiograms and electroencephalograms. Needless to say, numerous technological advances have occurred since the invention of the telegraph and telephone, such as increased broadband access and high-definition image capabilities, which make the possibilities for providing health care to remote locations even greater. Furthermore, two-way, live videoconferencing now allows patients, family practitioners, and specialists to instantaneously exchange information while it simultaneously enables health care providers to visualize images that are critical in evaluating, diagnosing, and treating patients. The ability to see visual cues and body language is also a critical factor in the treatment of psychiatric patients. Now, in addition to the fields of cardiology and psychiatry, many medical specialties are actively engaged in telemedicine including obstetrics, pediatrics, critical care, and radiology [1–4].

Telemedicine has also allowed access to care for those underserved populations where a shortage of specialists exists and where care may be limited by geographic distance. Technological advances such as these have prodded an increase in the utilization of telemedicine that we see today in over 50 specialty areas. Now, a myriad of services that traditionally only took place face-to-face are being conducted "virtually" and instantaneously. Consultations, medical procedures, examinations and assessments, educational programs, and research activities can now be performed from nearly anywhere as long as the technology exists in order to support it.

Telemedicine is usually delivered in two main ways—"store-and-forward" and "real-time" communication. "Store-and-forward" means that various types of medical information including images, diagnostic information, medical histories, and the like are prepared and then transferred electronically to another destination to be used or reviewed at a later time. This type of modality is commonly used in fields such as pathology and radiology and in cases where the medical issue is not of an urgent nature, especially where still pictures are important. With "real-time" tele-medicine, the same sort of medical information may be exchanged among individuals in different locations simultaneously and in "real time" without delay.

ENABLING ACCESS TO CARE

The capacity to reach beyond time and geographical constraints has far-reaching implications for both health care and research. The ultimate goal of research is to further an understanding of disease in order to improve treatment and improve the health of all. The most valid and reliable research results depend upon the ability to access all parts of a population, and are one of the hallmarks of comparative effectiveness research [5]. If certain segments of the population are not taken into account, then the results of the study will only be pertinent to that specific group of people. Encompassing a larger population ensures that the results are as accurate as possible and a greater likelihood exists that the results will be pertinent to the group under study. Examining multiple factors from a large sample enhances our understanding of the disease or condition. Because telemedicine enables access to remote areas and a greater number of people, it encourages valid and reliable results. The discoveries that are gleaned from research are then used to shape and guide standards of care to further promote quality health care, especially in underserved or rural populations. Telemedicine furthers this step in the process of translational research by adding to the validity and reliability of research results, which ultimately aids in the development of a consensus regarding what is considered "best practices."

With its ability to access remote areas and to facilitate communication over live videoconferencing to a large group of practitioners, telemedicine also serves as an ideal mode of delivery of best practices so that these practices can be implemented into patient care. Implementing standards of care in large institutions where practitioners have access to specialist consults and educational opportunities occurs more quickly than in rural areas where practitioners lack access to such resources. Therefore, a great need exists in these rural areas in terms of access to critical resources that guide clinical practice. Telemedicine enables access to resources in these underserved areas since it serves as a conduit for dialog and consultation in a multitude of ways.

Furthermore, it is becoming more widespread for education through teleconferencing for continuing professional development of physicians, nurses, and allied health personnel, also known as e-learning. E-learning has been shown to be as good as, if not better than, traditional instructor-led lectures in contributing to demonstrated learning, especially when interaction is encouraged. Telemedicine supports the interaction among specialists, primary-care physicians, other medical personnel, the patient and patient's family in addressing the needs of the patient, which increases understanding of the patient's condition and on-going care. Thus, systems of care are better coordinated and more informed decision-making on the part of all involved in the treatment plan can occur.

TELEMEDICINE CORE FACILITY

Telemedicine programs that aim to eliminate impediments to health care such as lack of access to resources in rural locations by making educational opportunities readily available through interactive educational videoconferences have been developed. Individuals and families that live in rural areas represent about 20% of the US population. In Arkansas, 61 of 75 counties are designated as medically underserved areas, with many of those counties facing health care provider shortages. For example, our center developed a Community-Based Research and Education (CoBRE) Core facility that was created to promote the translation of neuroscience applications from the clinic to the community, overcoming one of the T2 blocks to translational research. This infrastructure consists of the use of real-time, diagnostic quality telemedicine for research (design, planning, and conduction) and educational (training, dissemination, and implementation of research) purposes; the former to conduct research on community-based practices and public health initiatives, the latter to develop research projects, consensus guidelines, and common treatment strategies across diverse environments.

Successful telemedicine transmissions are achieved when broadband speeds approach a minimum of 384 kbps up/768 kbps down. Greater bandwidth allows for clearer connections with less movement artifact. Within University of Arkansas for Medical Sciences (UAMS), Center for Distance Health (CDH) telemedicine infrastructure, one of the largest state driven telemedicine networks within the United States, successful transmissions are achieved through a myriad of networks. Some hospitals are able to utilize point-to-point T1 trunk lines put in place by the Arkansas Department of Health where as others are using point-to-point T1 lines that run from UAMS through the CDH network. For video units placed on the UAMS and Arkansas Children's Hospital campus, the network is more than sufficient to meet these bandwidth demands internally. Other facilities are able to meet the bandwidth needs within their own internal network or by having business class broadband lines installed at their locations. This latter method of using a local Internet Service Provider (ISP) is very effective in smaller clinics or at a physician's residence where bandwidth is an issue, and it also alleviates any firewall concerns. In the era of cloud computing, still other organizations are moving away from point-to-point T1's and migrating to Multiprotocol Label Switching services provided by some of the larger ISP's, which helps to mitigate both the cost and support of maintaining a T1 circuit.

Once a site acquires the appropriate infrastructure for successful telemedicine transmission, the next step is to put in place the H.323 or Session Initiation Protocol (SIP) video devices to be used on the network. In rough terms, H.323 and SIP are protocols that allow for the transmission of video and audio across a network. While video devices should ideally all be using the same protocol, there are devices called gateways that can allow units using H.323, SIP, or telephone-based Integrated Services Digital Network to all communicate with one another. Equipment used to communicate via a specific protocol must be compatible with that network since different protocols do not communicate with each other. In cases where there are two different protocol devices that need to communicate with one another, a gateway is required to translate and then convert incoming and outgoing signals. Therefore, it is best and simplest when all sites involved in a conference obtain equipment configured the same way.

The actual videoconference units consist of a monitor with speakers, camera, microphone, and a codec. A codec or compression/decompression unit decompresses an incoming signal and then compresses the signals in order to translate it and send it out. A codec is to a videoconferencing unit what a PC is to a monitor and a keyboard. Units can be configured to serve as primarily clinical units or primarily educational units. A clinical unit can have its components mounted to a mobile cart so that the unit can be transported to various locations, including the patient's bedside, to various treatment provider workstations, and other points of service. Videoconferencing equipment can be connected to medical devices to transmit images using Video Graphics Array, *Digital Visual Interface*, Separate Video, *High-Definition Multimedia Interface*, and various other cable connection types. Peripheral medical devices can also be connected to the unit, such as ultrasound units, stethoscopes, otoscopes, laryngoscopes, endoscopes, and the like so that patient procedures can be viewed in real time. New types of medical equipment with compatibility that can be connected to a telemedicine unit are evolving and being developed every day.

Units used for educational purposes will contain the same components as the clinical units without the addition of the peripheral medical devices. Since the educational units are used to conduct seminars and conferences for larger audiences, this type of unit will usually be located in a conference room with a monitor or television mounted on a wall and the other equipment located in a cabinet. These units have the capability to hook up to various hardware systems that enable paper documents to be transmitted and shown from a screen. Smaller educational units for those who may want to participate in the videoconference from an office or practice setting may be located at one's desktop. As a side note, several manufacturers produce models of desktop videoconferencing units that already include camera, codec, speakers, and monitor all in one device for desktop use. All equipment in our network utilizes standards-based equipment that employs encryption software to meet all compliance rules and regulations.

A high-definition monitor along with a call speed at or above 768 kbps has the capability of receiving a true high-definition (HD) image, but this is dependent on the site at the other end having an HD camera as well as the 768 kbps line speed to send an HD image. Regardless of whether the unit is designated as clinical or educational, the same core components make up every videoconferencing unit. The units also benefit from a laptop linked to the Internet for acquisition of materials such as guidelines, providing input to the guidelines, downloading treatment-related protocols, and accessing the archives of previous conferences and can be connected to medical documentation (Electronic Health Records, Medical Imaging Systems and Lab Repositories) for viewing via the telemedicine connection with those systems that are not integrated into the provider networks.

The Pediatric Physician Learning and Collaborative Education (Peds PLACE, a telemedicine program described later in this chapter) program comprises many sites and is therefore considered "multisite conferencing." Typically, one video unit can only connect to one other site. However, some units allow for upgrades that allow connecting up to four sites. In contrast, a multipoint control unit (MCU) allows for multiple simultaneous connections. The UAMS CDH has the ability to simultaneously connect 300 participants over video. During a conference, the units are connected via the MCU and while content can be controlled from any one video participant, the conference at large is administrated and controlled by a video conferencing technician who accesses the web interface of the MCU. Each site signs in for real-time videoconferencing, and the conference is moderated by a video operations team. The screen layout is such that anywhere from 1 to 20 sites can be displayed on the screen at any one time. However, for a larger conference like Peds PLACE, the screen is configured so that all sites will only see the presenting site until the "Question and Answers" (Q&A) segment. During the "Q&A" segment, the screen layout becomes what is called "voice switched," which will make the site that is currently speaking full screen at all other sites. Receiving training in and practicing video etiquette is important for participants in a videoconference. Just as in a room full of people when more than one person speaks, it is difficult to understand what any one person is saying. The same is true with videoconferencing. For example, during the Peds PLACE videoconference the moderator can call on each site for their contributions or questions, and a participant at the site simply unmutes their microphone via a button on his or her remote control and speaks.

Although not an essential component to conducting a videoconference, supplemental software, such as Media site, WebEx, and Blackboard to name a few, enables participants who cannot attend the actual videoconference to be able to listen and observe. Media site is one-way communication and is not truly interactive. In order to be viewed, the content of the videoconference is sent to the Media site from which it is then broadcast. Users access the Media site by logging in via their personal computer. For educational purposes, continuing education is not earned when accessing conferences via a media site without supplemental questions since it is not a two-way communication device. However, Media site monitors those linked via the Web who provides written comments or questions. The written questions can be addressed by the participants at the conference, making the information available to the entire network. Therefore, access is not limited to those sites in which the units are located.

NEONATAL INTENSIVE CARE

Another major area of focus utilizing this Core Facility is "Tele-nursery" that was established for both educational and research purposes in the care of sick neonates including very low birth weight (VLBW) infants. "Tele-nursery" is a tri-weekly clinical and research program. The Tele-nursery program was initiated by placing telemedicine units with real-time video-conferencing and diagnostic quality imaging units in lower level nurseries linked to a level 3 nursery with a large academic practice. This telemedicine network linked the academic medical center with 24 community hospitals allowing live interactive videoconferencing. A 24-hour call center is also in place that is staffed by nurses with on-site physician access who provide case-management services for patients and their physicians for multiple CDH programs. Through simple, daily census and rounding administered through telemedicine, the telemedicine program can determine the best locations and most appropriate patients to transport. Through on-site telemedicine in nursery areas, especially in hospital nurseries without neonatology coverage, treatment options for high-risk neonates are reviewed in real time with pediatric subspecialists. In addition, other services such as coordination of discharge is accomplished with specialty nurses trained in discharge of high-risk neonates.

"Tele-nursery" works with the Antenatal Guidelines and Neonatal Educational Learning System (ANGELS), the obstetrical portion of the UAMS telemedicine program, to form a perinatal outreach program. VLBW births are a leading cause of death and disability in infants, major sources of stress for parents, and an economic burden for private and public health insurance programs. Delivery at hospitals offering specialized pre- and perinatal care is thought to be effective in improving birth outcomes and perhaps reducing medical costs. However, women residing in rural and underserved areas typically lack access to these centers, and perinatal and neonatal subspecialists who can assist community physicians with diagnosis and management of high-risk pregnancies and their neonates. The five main goals of this program are to (1) support practitioners in rural areas, (2) build relationships between these practitioners and pediatric specialists at the primary care center, (3) learn from the experience of these practitioners, (4) translate current research findings into useful advice and community health improvement, and (5) improve the health care of pregnant mothers and their children.

The Peds PLACE program develops, maintains, and disseminates a set of evidence-based clinical guidelines and protocols to support community caregivers caring for children. Additionally, case-based weekly educational conferences are broadcast in conjunction with the guidelines. These teleconferences employ state-of-the-art, real-time technologies, ensuring a high level of interaction between the speaker and the audience. The program addresses common disease management questions. Further, the guidelines developed are then published on the ANGELS Web site, which have become extremely popular on a national level. In addition, there are usually a number of international viewers across the United States, Europe, and India [6,7].

Another aspect of this program includes the assessment of outcomes. Delivery patterns, evaluated through a linked Medicaid database before and after the "Tele-nursery" initiative, found that VLBW neonates were transferred to higher level centers for delivery. This program demonstrated that telemedicine is an effective way to translate evidence-based medicine into clinical practice when combined with a weekly educational teleconference. Additionally, surveys reported that the electronic medium was as effective as in-person delivery among physicians for continuing education among physicians and nurses. The study suggested that telemedicine-based education and consultation combined with guideline dissemination can be effective in enhancing access to beneficiary specialty care for the management of high-risk pregnancies, particularly for rural and underserved populations [8]. In doing so, these approaches may facilitate the development of regionalized centers of perinatal care that improve access and health outcomes of VLBW infants.

Through Peds PLACE, a number of other studies have been initiated. One study entitled, "Continuing Professional Development Through Telemedicine: An Assessment of Peds PLACE," aimed to assess to what extent Peds PLACE was meeting its goal of aiding in professional development, ultimately resulting in the implementation of best practices into the community. With over 500 participants, the results demonstrated a high degree of satisfaction with Peds PLACE and considered it an effective way to address the continuing education needs of health care personnel throughout the state, especially in rural and underserved areas. Future studies will address if learning is taking place, at first by inserting questions at key points to maintain attention and check for learning, later assessing learning to determine if behavior is being changed (how health care is delivered), and lastly to evaluate if outcomes are improving as a result.

EMERGENCY DEPARTMENTS

On the basis of the success of this program, the existing CoBRE was expanded to establish a similar program called Emergency Department Physician Learning and Collaborative Education (EDs PLACE), a statewide emergency medicine network through which translational research projects can be implemented via telemedicine initiatives. The launch of EDs PLACE was also in response to the 2006 Institute of Medicine (IOM) report on the future of emergency care, which advocated for measures to evaluate emergency care research (ECR) needs and address gaps [9]. Similar to Peds PLACE, the purpose of this ECR program was to address disparities in rural health care and to determine methods to improve education, communication, and consultation with rural emergency departments (EDs) in order to improve health care. EDs PLACE links 15 EDs located across Arkansas. The ultimate aim of this program is to improve health care and to cut costs through fostering collaboration and communication between UAMS, an academic health center, and the health care providers at community EDs. The aim is that these partnerships utilizing research will improve the effectiveness of community EDs.

An assumption inherent to the practice of emergency medicine is that rapid diagnoses and timely interventions for acute illness or disease improve patient outcomes. The vast majority of illnesses or injuries evaluated in the ED are time-dependent and time-sensitive in terms of their diagnosis, and treatment and resources such as imaging technology or specialty consults are available to ED patients on an around-the-clock basis. Therefore, ECR aims to evaluate emergent care delivery in order to advance patient care. Participants at an ECR network conference defined ECR as "the systematic examination of patient care that should be continuously available to diverse populations presenting with undifferentiated symptoms of acute illness, injury, or acutely decompensated chronic illness, and whose outcomes depend on timely diagnosis and treatment" [10].

Therefore, the scope of ECR encompasses not only the processes that occur within the ED visit itself, but also the overall system of emergency care delivery. Critical components of the system consist of prehospital care or the various settings of the patient prior to the ED visit, access to care including transportation modalities, short-term outcomes of the ED visit in terms of inpatient hospitalizations, transfers or discharges, and ultimately long-term outcomes such as discharges to home, rehabilitation services, or other managed care services. Examining the dynamics of these parts of the system aids in a better understanding of the process and effectiveness of patient care in the ED.

Another overarching component to the system of emergency care is time. Because time is critical in emergency care, tracking the duration of each of these phases and its effects on other aspects of the system is important in assessing the effectiveness and impact of the overall system and also in understanding short falls or gaps in patient care. The correlation of time with determining diagnoses, treatments/interventions, or optimal outcomes for the patient illuminates the workings of the system. Also essential to timely care is the rapid exchange of information. Therefore, the transfer and linkage of electronic data for research purposes among the various potential phases of care are crucial to successful research. EDs PLACE aims to address and evaluate all of these critical components to the emergency care system in order to benefit the way that treatment is developed and practiced.

CONCLUSION

Telemedicine enables effective community-based research by narrowing the gap between the patient population and health care provider that has been caused by distance, lack of resources, and/or lack of access. In doing so, telemedicine has brought critical components of health care delivery into awareness that need to be evaluated in order to develop, disseminate, and implement best practices of health care. Furthermore, new technologies are being developed, which will serve to further expand the possibilities for translational research that has the capability to greatly impact and promote health care for all.

REFERENCES

1. Lowery C, Bronstein J, McGhee J, Ott R, Reece EA, Mays GP. (2007) ANGELS and University of Arkansas for Medical Sciences paradigm for distant obstetrical care delivery. Am J Obstet Gynecol 196(6), 534.e1–9.
2. Hall-Barrow J, Hall RW, Burke BL, Jr. (2009a) Telemedicine and neonatal regionalization of care - ensuring that the right baby gets to the right nursery. Pediatr Ann 38, 557–561.
3. Marcin JP, Ellis J, Mawis R, Nagrampa E, Nesbitt TS, Dimand RJ. (2004) Using telemedicine to provide pediatric subspecialty care to children with special health care needs in an underserved rural community. [see comment]. Pediatrics 113, 1–6.
4. Hilty DM, Yellowlees PM, Nesbitt TS. (2006) Evolution of telepsychiatry to rural sites: changes over time in types of referral and in primary care providers' knowledge, skills and satisfaction. Gen Hosp Psychiatry 28, 367–373.
5. Whicher DM, Chalkidou K, Dhalla IA, Levin L, Tunis S. (2009) Comparative effectiveness research in Ontario, Canada: producing relevant and timely information for health care decision makers. Milbank Q 87, 585–606.
6. Hall RW, Hall-Barrow J, Garcia-Rill E. (2010) Neonatal regionalization through telemedicine using a community-based research and education core facility. Ethn Dis 20, S1-136–S1-140.

7. Hall-Barrow J, Hall RW, Burke BL, Jr. (2009b) Telemedicine and neonatal regionalization of care—ensuring that the right baby gets to the right nursery. Pediatr Ann 38, 557–561.

8. Gonzalez-Espada WJ, Hall-Barrow J, Hall RW, Burke BL, Smith CE. (2009) Peds PLACE: quality continuing medical education in Arkansas. J Ark Med Soc 105, 211–213.

9. Mark Courtney D, Neumar RW, Venkatesh AK, Kaji AH, Cairns CB, Lavonas E, Richardson LD. (2009) Unique characteristics of emergency care research: scope, populations, and infrastructure. Acad Emerg Med 16, 990–994.

10. Whicher DM, Chalkidou K, Dhalla IA, Levin L, Tunis S. (2009) Comparative effectiveness research in Ontario, Canada: producing relevant and timely information for health care decision makers. Milbank Q 87, 585–606.

10 Implications for the Future

Edgar Garcia-Rill

The last of the elements impeding the progress of translational research that we have not discussed are fragmented infrastructure and incompatible databases. These obstacles can be overcome, although not without some investment. Such investments are necessary to the future of both basic and translational science, and we will address the benefits gained from investment in translational neuroscience research. Finally, we will discuss a model for formally restructuring the interactions between clinical and basic science departments at academic health centers in order to promote more translational neuroscience research.

FRAGMENTED INFRASTRUCTURE

The issues related to fragmented infrastructure were partly addressed in the chapter on Core Facilities and their design. The former Clinical Translational Science Award (CTSA), now called National Center for Advancing Translational Science (NCATS), program encouraged the location of these facilities within a single institute or center, precisely to avoid the scattered facility syndrome. Centralization of resources is more economical and convenient for investigators and patients. Which types of equipment are included obviously depends on the expertise of the investigators in the institute or center for translational neuroscience research. Throughout this book, we discuss the potential types of Core Facilities that can be established, and ours is only a short list of the possibilities. By now it should be evident that translational research has many faces and many avenues. However, it is clear that the technology in the brain sciences needs new approaches. For example, the more and more detailed visualization provided by higher and higher power magnetic resonance imagings at greater and greater cost is producing little agreement and not advancing therapeutic strategies. While these techniques remain incredibly valuable for diagnostic procedures, they have yet to provide consensus guidelines for

Translational Neuroscience: A Guide to a Successful Program, First Edition. Edited by Edgar Garcia-Rill.
© 2012 John Wiley & Sons, Inc. Published 2012 by John Wiley & Sons, Inc.

treatment. Part of the problem stems from the use of individualized measurement algorithms, so that comparisons across institutions are difficult at best. The field of neuroimaging needs to develop optimized and standardized methods that allow comparisons across institutions. Only then can the massive investment already made in this technology begin to make a greater impact on health and cost savings.

In addition, while these images are impressive, they say little of the real-time activity of the central nervous system. As discussed previously, new approaches to disseminating techniques that detect brain function in real time are much needed. The use of magnetoencephalography (MEG) has been neglected by US funding agencies to the point that major manufacturers in Canada and the United States have been forced to close their doors. Europe is far ahead of the United States in MEG technology, and stands to make significant headway in dissecting the online workings of the brain. The clinical applications of this technology are proven in some areas, for example, in epilepsy surgery, in which the diagnosis of the disorder, plots of the eloquent (healthy) tissue, and of the initial ictal (seizure) event all are reimbursable by insurers. Such information is critical to performing optimal surgical resection of ictal tissue, and preventing follow-up surgeries representing a safer (healthy tissue is less likely to be removed) and less costly (prevent additional surgery) approach. For research purposes, however, this technology stands to suffer from similar problems as the imaging industry, as long as protocols and algorithms are not optimized and standardized.

INCOMPATIBLE DATABASES

The US health care system invests almost $2 trillion annually yet the system is inefficient and of poor quality in too many areas. In general, providers lack the information systems necessary to coordinate a patient's care with other providers, to share needed information, to monitor compliance with best-practice guidelines, and to measure and improve performance. Some industries have lowered costs and improved quality through investments in information technology. Health care could achieve similar results if a serious effort is made toward compatible databases [1]. While curing the health care system is beyond the range of translational neuroscience, the accomplishments of such research would be multiplied if these incompatibilities were addressed.

For example, implementation of integrated data sources, including patient electronic medical records, decision support systems, and computerized order entry for medications would provide rapid access to patient information that could coordinate health information with other providers, patients, and insurers. Dramatic savings would be realized in the form of reduced hospital stays (due to better scheduling and coordination), reduced administrative time, and produce efficient drug utilization. Such systems would increase safety by providing immediate information to physicians, for example, about potential adverse reactions with a patient's other drugs. Proper information technology would help with prevention by scanning patient records for risk factors and by recommending appropriate preventive services, such as vaccinations and screenings. Patients using remote monitoring systems could transmit their vital signs from their homes to the providers, allowing a rapid response to problems. Effective disease management could reduce the need for hospitalization, thereby improving both health and reducing costs [1]. In the telemedicine chapter, we saw how this technology can make an impact in reducing infant mortality, saving lives, and decreasing costs due to complications like intraventricular hemorrhage, all with rather modest investment. The costs of implementing an information technology health care system are high, but the potential improvement in care would better outcomes, the increased savings would far outweigh the initial investment, and the long-term savings would be significant enough to help reduce our investment in health care.

Why is this important for translational research? Because, aside from helping achieve the ultimate goal of improving the health of our citizens, such a system would provide a gold mine of information for assessing effectiveness and costs. This aspect of translational research could decrease costs even without implementing a national health information system. Comparative effectiveness research (CER) is designed to inform health care decisions by providing evidence on the effectiveness, benefits, and harms of different treatment options. The evidence is generated from research studies that compare drugs, medical devices, tests, surgeries, or ways to deliver health care. Researchers assess the evidence about the benefits and harms of each choice for different groups of people from existing clinical trials, clinical studies, and other research. Investigators also conduct studies that generate new evidence of effectiveness of a test, treatment, procedure, or health care service. CER requires the development, expansion, and use of a variety of data sources and methods to conduct relevant research and disseminate the results in a form that is usable by clinicians, patients, policy-makers, and health plans and other payers. Interestingly, pharmaceutical and medical device companies have been accused of quietly working to neutralize the impact of CER, while superficially embracing the concept [2]. This tactic involves undercutting efforts to actually use such research or other technology assessment tools, including cost-effectiveness, to change the practice of medicine.

The answer to such an effort is to "defeat them with excellence." There is little doubt that we must cut health care spending, at the risk of spending too much of our GNP on just staying alive. Translational neuroscience CER can help tremendously in determining, for example, if the therapeutic effects of certain drugs (say, psychoactive agents) are really better than placebo, or better than generic versions of the same agent. Many pharmaceutical companies discourage the use of generics in the name of safety, but it could be in the name of the profit motive [3]. We need to establish scientifically if such safety claims are true. This is not a simple issue since there are examples, for instance, in epilepsy treatment, in which the use of certain generics can lead to serious side effects for patients being treated on specific antiseizure medication. Another example where CER can help is in the study of slightly altered drugs. A standard strategy of some drug companies is to develop a "long-acting" version of the same drug near the end of patent protection of the original agent. Are these really "better," or are they just driving up the cost of health care? The opportunities for research, and for optimizing health care while maintaining efficacy and safety, are enormous and should be undertaken by unbiased investigators. The Agency for Health Research and Quality, along with Federal and state Medicare agencies fund the bulk of CER. Increased funding for their efforts are paramount if we are to control health care costs. Every well-designed study has the potential to improve health and cut costs.

THE BENEFITS OF TRANSLATIONAL RESEARCH

What was the time frame for translational implementation of basic discoveries before this newly found drive that has grown over the last 5–10 years? An interesting study up to the year 2000, of the lag time between the first description of an intervention and its initial application to humans was found to be ~24 years (range 14–44 years) [4]. The lag time was decreased for interventions that were not later refuted, so that the lag time for those was ~16 years (range 4–50 years). These authors suggested that multidisciplinary collaborations on new interventions are essential, that proof of effectiveness requires large randomized clinical trials, and that translational efforts on old diseases need novel agents and technology [4]. These are precisely the guiding principles behind the design of translational research efforts over the last decade. Hopefully, a similar study conducted 5–10 years from now will show that these lag times have been significantly decreased by our efforts in translational neuroscience. If so, funding for translational research efforts will need to be increased; if not, a reassessment of our approach will be required.

If we do not yet know if translational research will pay off, why fund it? The old adage goes, "If you think research is expensive, try disease." The economic cost of illness in the year 2000 was $3 trillion, about 31% of the nation's GNP at that time. This figure takes into account the "direct" costs of illness that refers to the actual medical costs of treatment and procedures needed to manage a disease, as well as the "indirect" costs that refer to the cost associated with loss of productivity and ability to work due to illness [2]. Past advances in research have significantly reduced the costs associated with diseases such as schizophrenia, tuberculosis, and peptic ulcers. In addition, in the mid-1990s, new treatments for AIDS that were in part generated by federally funded research enabled millions of people to return to work and ultimately reduced indirect costs by 60% [2]. Furthermore, according to one study, death rates from cardiovascular disease have declined by approximately 50% since 1970. One-third of this reduction is a result of developments in medical technology [2].

In addition, health care costs are likely to increase in the future. In 1970, 9.7% of the population was 65 years or older. The current rate is approximately 12.4%, and in 2030 the rate is predicted to be 19.8% [3]. Moreover, infectious illnesses continue to emerge and increase health care spending. Despite future increased health care costs, the National Institutes of Health (NIH) health care budget allotment for medical research has fallen from 2.2% of GNP in 1980 to 1.6% in 2000. This trend is concerning due to an impending rise in health care costs. Investing in research is the only way in which these costs will be mitigated through greater medical advances that will help prevent and treat such illnesses. In light of this, the question of whether not to fund research becomes moot. Instead, the focus needs to revolve around ways to increase investment in research. In the meantime, universities can lay the groundwork for the conditions that will facilitate translational research.

THE RESHAPING OF BASIC SCIENCE DEPARTMENTS

In recent years, there has been a trend to reorganize. Departments of Anatomy, Physiology, Pharmacology, etc., were in some cases coalesced into a single Department of Neuroscience or Neurobiology. Other departments like Immunology, Microbiology, and Biochemistry have been merged into Cell Biology or Molecular Biology departments. Such reorganizations typically follow the basic science research strengths of a particular institution. However, there are always faculty members who find themselves in the "wrong" department. For example, a molecular/cell biologist neuroscientist may find little interactions with systems-based scientists in a Neuroscience department, or with hard-core molecular biologists in a Molecular Biology department. Other institutions have gone the way of mega departments, lumping all or most of these into Departments of Biomedical Sciences. Most of these changes have been touted as essential to enhance research productivity. In many cases, monetary considerations are behind these changes, mainly designed to save administrative and personnel costs. Graduate programs have followed suit, so that graduate students are shuttled into "generic" "biomedical science" tracks for their initial training, from which they then split off into their area of interest. These approaches are excellent for students who do not know what area of research they want to work in, or for those who already know, but it is not neuroscience. The curricula of these biomedical science programs have little or no basic neuroscience in the first year, which makes graduate degrees in neuroscience unfairly longer than the other tracks. Graduate programs that include early neuroscience training should garner more informed graduate trainees.

Some institutions have gone from department- or discipline-based organizations to center- or disease-based structures, such as cancer centers, diabetes institutes, aging centers, and the like. These structures help coalesce like-minded scientists, but also suffer from limits imposed by the label placed on an individual's research, sometimes making the flexibility needed for translational research more difficult. So, what is the best organizational plan for promoting translational neuroscience research while maintaining solid basic science accomplishments yet enabling clinician scientist training? In order to answer that question, we need to determine what is required to establish a successful translational neuroscience research program.

The first requirement is institutional commitment. The academic health center needs to make an investment of time and money to establish translational research. Second, it should develop an institution-wide mentoring program for young faculty, both basic and clinical. Third, it must identify the most appropriate leader for such a task. Institutions with a CTSA typically identify someone who can lead the clinical research infrastructure, but in many cases these busy clinician scientists can handle the demands of a CTSA, but a program in translational research needs more than a CTSA can offer. The ideal leader is an individual with considerable research experience, solid mentoring experience, and an unselfish attitude toward building the program. In order to gain the trust and cooperation of clinical chairs, established mentors, and young clinician scientists, this leader needs to be able to speak the same language and to have their best interests at heart. This individual does not necessarily need to be a clinician scientist, in fact, senior basic science researchers with mature careers and deep knowledge of applied science are well suited to this role. An established basic scientist with a track record of productivity is just as likely to gain the respect and cooperation of clinical chairs. These chairs understand that, if they are to recruit and retain their research-oriented faculty, they must provide the release time required to establish an active laboratory. Someone who has done precisely that and is willing to share their time and knowledge with young clinician scientists represents an excellent ally to the clinical chairs. Considering the demands on their time on a daily basis, a clinician with a busy practice may be more difficult to find as a leader than a basic scientist who has more flexibility in scheduling the demands of growing such a program.

Experience in mentoring, and all it entails as discussed in Chapter 2, is a prerequisite for such a role. The demands on the leader's time by a group of young clinician scientists, who themselves can only meet on a restricted or off-hour schedule, can be considerable. Possessing the characteristic of an altruistic nature is paramount, given the complex and time-consuming interactions being forged. Senior basic science researchers have typically gained much experience in mentoring of their postdoctoral fellows, graduate, and other students working in their labs. They have nurtured these trainees in many of the same tasks that young clinician scientists with limited research experience will need. In addition, experience in human subject research is essential considering the many pitfalls embodied in gaining approval and conducting research on human subjects. This is perhaps the most time-consuming area for young clinician scientists, and their success is predicated on making their way through the regulatory process while learning the requirements but not being unduly delayed. This task is greatly facilitated by mentors who do have experience in human subject research, who can help frame the protocols, and who can steer them through the system. In some cases, multiple mentors may be needed if a clinical investigator is bridging very basic technology, animal models, and research on humans. The ability of the program leader and/or mentor to train the young scientist in collaboration with the mentor will be critical in advancing a successful research career.

Most institutions have precisely this kind of leader in their basic science departments. By forging an alliance, through these established and willing faculty members, between the basic and clinical departments, academic health centers can build a successful translational research program with existing personnel. That is, the initial development of such a program may require little to no expenditure. Forward-thinking basic science chairs realize that such alliances are highly desirable. The separation between basic and clinical departments in some medical schools has grown as basic science departments become more and more esoteric in their cell biology or molecular biology research, distancing themselves from the more proximal demands of clinical practice. A formalized alliance between basic science and clinical departments would help bridge that gap, and build the research infrastructure of the institution. Many faculty members in basic science departments can certainly benefit from a more informed attitude about clinical medicine. Those most willing to learn will find the opportunities to grow research programs parallel to their own successful programs. The contributions from basic science faculty with experience in a host of areas will help a translational research program immensely, from the expertise provided on techniques to writing talent to simply managing a laboratory. Successful basic research faculty will be absolutely essential to building an effective translational research program.

Some institutions or departments may want to stimulate such interactions by informally organizing researchers into magnet areas, however, this approach will be slow and interrupted by individual priorities. Without formalizing the program with a mandated structure, progress will be vicarious, while creating a center or institute under the umbrella of the research arm of the institution will speed collaborations and help stimulate the generation of joint projects and grant applications. By creating a center or division of translational neuroscience, an institution can set up an alliance between relevant clinical and basic science departments. For example, a department of Neuroscience can form a translational neuroscience research initiative in collaboration with such departments as Neurology, Neurosurgery, and Psychiatry, as well as elements of Pediatrics, Otolaryngology, and Physical Medicine and Rehabilitation. Not all faculty members in a department need to be involved, only those who are committed to building their respective research programs. Given such alliances, funding for jump-starting such an effort could be more easily negotiated with the institution, especially if the departments contribute in terms of release time and even funding. Such an initiative can begin modestly by using existing facilities and providing pilot study money for willing scientists. However, it is clear that a considerable investment needs to be made in just the right kind of Core Facilities and just the right sort of personnel. Chapter 3 describes some of the types of Cores that could serve such an initiative, while other chapters provide detailed descriptions of only a few areas of translational neuroscience research that can be pursued. Moreover, the most important but perhaps most costly element is the release time from clinical duties for clinician scientists. The trend toward incorporating research rotations in medical school and residency programs is growing, so that providing appropriate research time for young faculty is just the logical next step. With the help of experienced leaders in the basic and clinical sciences working together for the benefit of the institution (and not necessarily any one department), we can nurture the next generation of translational neuroscientists. It is for them to see that the advances we make reach our constituents to improve health care.

Given the doubling of the NIH budget, the sequencing of the human genome, and the solid scientific advances in basic biology over the past 20 years, we are poised to translate these advances into clinical medicine to alleviate suffering from disease. Every institution can contribute to the implementation of translational research programs. While national level initiatives can begin the process and facilitate implementation by providing funding, disseminating information, and streamlining cumbersome regulatory processes, academic health centers can have a greater impact in gaining public support at the local level for translational research, to begin to establish the infrastructure, and to train the workforce of the future. A well-planned and formulated translational research initiative will pay enormous dividends in terms of grant funding, good will, and improvements in the health of our citizens.

REFERENCES

1. Rand Corporation; Health Information Technology. (2005) Can HIT lower costs and improve quality? http://www.rand.org/pubs/research_briefs/RB9136/index1.html.

2. Bartlett Foote S; The Hastings Center. (2011) How comparative effectiveness research can save money. http://healthcarecostmonitor.thehastingscenter.org/suasanbartlettfoote/how-comparative-effectiveness-research-can-save-money/.
3. Fitzhugh M. (2011) The Burrill Report. Senate panel criticizes Sanofi tactics to delay competition. http://www.burrillreport.com/article-3538.html.
4. Contopoulos-Ioannidis DG, Alexiou GA, Gouvias TC, Ioannidis JPA. (2008) Life cycle of translational research for medical interventions. Science 321, 1298–1299.

Index